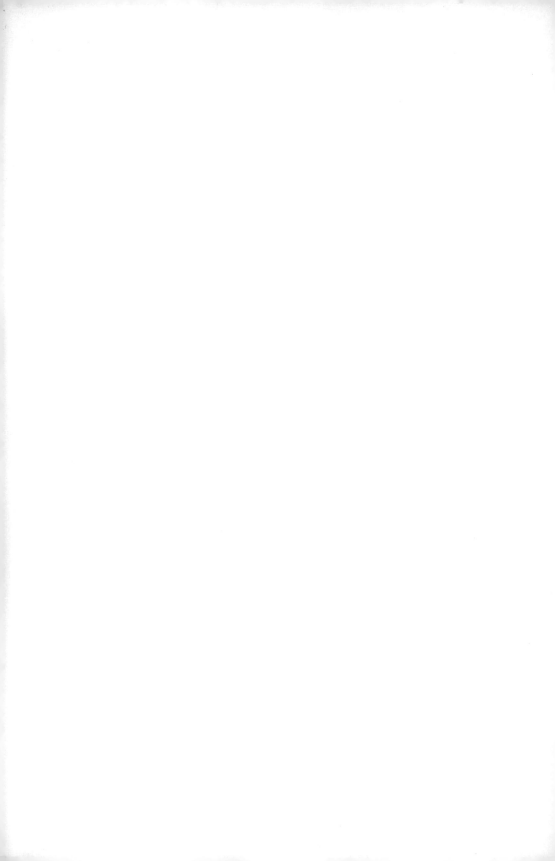

PHYSICIANS' HANDBOOK
OF NUTRITIONAL
SCIENCE

THE IMPORTANCE OF PRENATAL NUTRITION

In January of 1972 and shortly thereafter the American Medical Association placed identical full page advertisements in many large newspapers and prominent weekly magazines. Most of the full page was filled by a picture of a pregnant woman. Beneath the picture was this very significant statement:

The time to start feeding your baby right is several years before it's born.

By the time you've started to knit things, it could already be too late.

To nurture the baby growing inside her, a mother needs the strength that comes from years of good eating habits. During pregnancy, nutrition can have a direct, permanent effect on early brain growth. A seriously malnourished mother means a seriously deprived fetus. And that means a child born with less than full potential, physically and mentally.

Sound scary? It is. A malnourished mother is more likely to bear a premature, undersized baby (and the younger she is, the greater is the risk). The kind of baby who is least equipped to cope with the demands of living in today's society. The kind of baby who suffers the highest infant mortality rate.

Actually, the rate of infant mortality *has* improved in the U.S. It has dropped 25 percent in 10 years.

But more can be done. Much more. *If* society can be educated and motivated to better dietary habits. *Then* we can break a link in the vicious circle of poverty and ignorance that leads to malnutrition . . . that leads to underdeveloped children . . . that leads to poverty and ignorance again.

A big part of the job is education. We at the American Medical Association want to do our part. (70 percent of our budget goes to health and scientific education.)

One of the things the AMA will be doing in this area is to sponsor the National Congress on the Quality of Life, March 22-25 in Chicago. We hope it will be an important step in reaching this basic health standard for America: a *healthy mother* and a *healthy child*.

With all of man's concern about his environment, we doctors want to remind him of his first and most formative environment. The mother's womb.

America's Doctors of Medicine

PHYSICIANS' HANDBOOK
OF NUTRITIONAL
SCIENCE

By

ROGER J. WILLIAMS, Ph.D., D.Sc.

Clayton Foundation, Biochemical Institute
Department of Chemistry
The University of Texas
Austin, Texas

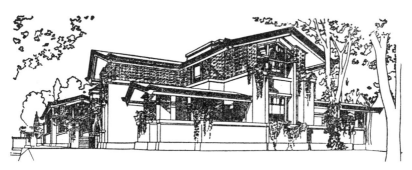

CHARLES C THOMAS • PUBLISHER
Springfield • Illinois • U.S.A.

Publication Number 963
AMERICAN LECTURE SERIES®

A Monograph in
The BANNERSTONE DIVISION *of*
AMERICAN LECTURES IN LIVING CHEMISTRY

Edited by
I. NEWTON KUGELMASS, M.D., Ph.D., Sc.D.
Consultant to the Departments of Health and Hospitals
New York City

Published and Distributed Throughout the World by
CHARLES C THOMAS · PUBLISHER
Bannerstone House
301-327 East Lawrence Avenue, Springfield, Illinois, U.S.A.

© *1975 by* CHARLES C THOMAS · PUBLISHER
ISBN 0-398-03256-4
Library of Congress Catalog Card Number, 74-9884

With THOMAS BOOKS *careful attention is given to all details of
manufacturing and design. It is the Publisher's desire to present books
that are satisfactory as to their physical qualities and artistic possibilities
and appropriate for their particular use.* THOMAS BOOKS *will be true
to those laws of quality that assure a good name and good will.*

Printed in the United States of America
Y-2

Library of Congress Cataloging in Publication Data

Williams, Roger John, 1893-
    Physicians' handbook of nutritional science.

    (American lecture series, publication no. 963. A monograph in the
Bannerstone division of American lectures in living chemistry.)
    1. Nutrition. I. Title. [DNLM: 1. Nutrition. QU145 W276p]
TX353.W54   641.1   74-9884
ISBN 0-398-03256-4

FOREWORD

O UR LIVING CHEMISTRY SERIES was conceived by Editor and Publisher to advance the newer knowledge of chemical medicine
in the cause of clinical practice. The interdependence of chemistry
and medicine is so great that physicians are turning to chemistry and
chemists to medicine in order to understand the underlying basis of
life processes in health and disease. Once chemical truths, proofs and
convictions become sound foundations for clinical phenomena, key
hybrid investigators clarify the bewildering panorama of biochemical
progress for application in everyday practice, stimulation of experimental research, and extension of postgraduate instruction. Each of
our monographs thus unravels the chemical mechanisms and clinical
management of many diseases that have remained relatively static in
the minds of medical men for three thousand years. Our new Series
is charged with the *nisus élan* of chemical wisdom, supreme in choice
of international authors, optimal in standards of chemical scholar-
ship, provocative in imagination for experimental research, comprehensive in discussions of scientific medicine, and authoritative in
chemical perspective of human disorders.

Dr. Williams of Austin, Texas, gives clinicians a postgraduate perspective in everyday nutrition for everyday patients, well or sick. It
is a remarkable crystallization of crucial facts, not opinions, that will
stand the test of time. It is a vivid analysis of the effect of food and
its constituents on the human body. It is a clinical application of nutritional science to the health problems of young and old. The problems are always the same but the solutions differ with each individual,
and the author is a master of biochemical individuality. Every individual reveals a personal story of his own nutrition subject to modification for optimal health for optimal longevity by the principles
elucidated in this work by a great authority, not a scribe, an early
pioneer in the vitamins indispensable in cellular metabolism.

Man is what he eats. He cannot think well, work well, play well, love well, sleep well if he has not eaten well. The whole of nature is a conjugation of the verb to eat, in the active and passive, but the three meals must be adequate and balanced. Nutrition cannot be viewed only in relation to absence, deficiency, or excessive nutrients, for subtle physiological variations make marked differences in individuals and in states of mind in the same individual at different times. The personal practice of scientific nutrition contributes to the advance of peoples throughout the world, toward longer and more secure living, relatively free of disease and retarded mental and physical development. The food we eat and do not eat determines the calibre of health.

Optimal nutrition is essential for effective organ development and function; for normal reproduction, growth and maintenance; for optimum activity and working efficiency; for resistance to infection; for increased capacity to repair bodily damage or injury. We have come to a conception of nutritional health and disease by which the two merge into each other. And achieving and/or preserving the health of the body is easy to do without destroying the health of the mind. Life is not living, but living in health. Unfortunately, we are not sensible of the most perfect health as we are of the least sickness. Once understanding of Williams' nutrition is clear, eating is made easy without perpetual anxiety about good nutrition.

"For 99% of the time that man has been on Earth, he was a food gatherer

And only during the remaining 1% has he been a food producer

—natural and artificial."

I. Newton Kugelmass, M.D., Ph.D., Sc.D., *Editor*

PREFACE

IF THIS BOOK could be adequately described in the preface, it would not have been worth writing. It is designed primarily for the physician who wants to get "on top" of the subject of nutrition so that henceforth he will have no occasion to be apologetic when the subject is mentioned.

There has been a demand for this book on the part of physicians, and it has been written at their specific request. They have wished for something as straightforward, simple and concise as possible. Accordingly, in order to tell a coherent, comprehensible story, extensive discussions including qualifying complications are not included. Notes at the ends of chapters, however, give readers sources of further and more detailed information.

One of the important qualifications which must be possessed by a book for physicians is that it be scientifically sound and carefully discriminate between fact and fiction. While on occasion the author has presented his opinions, they are labelled as such. The main thrust of the book is to present *facts* from which the physician can draw his own deductions.

This is not a book of menus, recipes and diets. Nutrition, in the sense that thoroughgoing students must think of it, cannot be analyzed in terms of lettuce, tomatoes, beefsteak and beans. If it is to be dealt with scientifically, it must be outlined in far more fundamental terms.

This little volume is not concerned with what to tell your patients about nutrition. Physicians and those with the basic essentials of medical training are alone in a position to appreciate the nuances of nutrition as they appear today. Laymen are able to appreciate that nutrition is vitally important, and as patients they must be dealt with intelligently and sympathetically, but without training in physiology and biochemistry these patients are not able to grasp the full meaning of a sophisticated approach.

This book is not a catalogue of nutrients which may serve as potential "medicines" for the treatment of various diseased conditions. Nutrients sometimes appear to act like specific medicines, but as we shall see in later discussions their mode of action is different from that of drugs; to miss this fact is to miss much of the essence of nutritional science.

The main objective of this book can be summed up as follows: it is the author's ambitious hope that after reading this book the physician may be inclined to say to himself, "Now, for the first time, I really appreciate the deep significance and meaning of nutrition and its importance in medical practice."

ACKNOWLEDGMENTS

THE WRITING OF THIS BOOK was accomplished within a period of six months, but not without efficient and most appreciated help from many others. My immediate co-workers, Drs. James D. Heffley, Donald R. Davis, Man-Li Yew and Charles W. Bode all helped immeasurably by numerous encouraging consultations and valuable suggestions. Because of my eyesight difficulties Dr. Heffley took on largely the responsibility for the bibliography and the index. My colleagues in the Clayton Foundation Biochemical Institute, particularly Professors William Shive, Lester J. Reed, Robert E. Eakin and Daniel M. Ziegler also read portions of the manuscript both critically and sympathetically. Professor Shive took a special interest in Chapter 4, "What Are the Basic Principles Underlying Nutritional Science?", which he thought unusually important.

Regarding this chapter (4), I also consulted perhaps a score of outside authorities whom I will not name individually, because such a listing could be misleading and omissions from the list would almost surely be misinterpreted. Suffice it to say that the individuals consulted were for the most part prominent scientists and that their approval, after a few modifications, approached unanimity.

Mr. S. Rodman Thompson did some valuable library work and much of the typing and my associate, Mrs. Marguerite M. Biesele, supervised the preparation of the entire manuscript and gave much other expert help. My wife, M. Phyllis Williams, exerted her usual common sense and confident encouragement.

To all these people I express my heartfelt thanks for helping make this book possible.

ROGER J. WILLIAMS
Austin, Texas, 1974

CONTENTS

PHYSICIANS' HANDBOOK
OF NUTRITIONAL
SCIENCE

CHAPTER 1

THE ENVIRONMENTAL PROBLEM

IT IS A WELL-KNOWN FACT in biology that organisms in general, as they appear on earth, face what in some respects is an unfriendly environment. A newborn infant may need help in getting air into its lungs, and it certainly must be protected against the vagaries of the weather if it is to survive. Very early it must have a healthy mother, or a substitute to furnish it food.

We human beings have faced and struggled with environmental problems as long as we have existed—obtaining shelter, protection, warmth and suitable food.

In the last few years, since about 1970, the public has awakened to the fact that there is such a thing as the environment—something that requires watching, guarding and maintaining. Before this time there were very few magazine articles on the subject; now there are hundreds every year. Before this time, governmental allotments for environmental control were practically nonexistent; in 1972 Congress passed an environmental control bill involving about 25 billion dollars, particularly for water pollution control.

This tremendous upsurge of interest in the environment is the basis for the demand for this book. Physicians realize that the food we eat is a part of our external environment; like the air we breathe and the water we drink, food needs careful and intelligent scrutiny.

The problem of the environment is far from simple when considered in its entirety. Not only do our bodies demand (1) a suitable ambient temperature, (2) air to furnish oxygen, and (3) fluid to furnish water, but also (4) suitable fuels for sources of energy, and (5) "maintenance chemicals"—a whole gamut of biochemicals that need to be supplied regularly so that the metabolic machinery

3

can be built and kept in working order.

The food-energy needs of the human race have often been the subject of discussion and calculation. Where to get this energy for an expanding population is a real question, and many discussions have centered around the problem of how to get more energy-yielding food from each acre or square mile of the earth's land and water surface.

Little detailed attention has been paid in these discussions to the very real need on the part of human beings for the maintenance chemicals referred to above—the chemicals we need to take in daily in order that we can continue to metabolize food and utilize fuel.

It is interesting to note that some organisms, notably such insects as houseflies and honeybees, are biologically built so that during their short adult life span they can live on essentially pure sugar and require practically no maintenance chemicals such as we have included under our item number 5 above. If adult human beings were built like houseflies or honeybees, the problem of their nutrition would be indeed a simple one, and heavy sugar cane crops could fill all our nutritional needs. Actually a close look at housefly or honeybee nutrition reveals that during the larval stage of their development these organisms require a good supply of the same sort of maintenance chemicals that we human beings need. The difference is that these insects, once they have their metabolic machinery built, require little or no further maintenance, whereas human beings certainly do, not only during their prolonged developmental period but during adulthood also.

The problem of the maintenance chemicals needed by human beings cannot be disposed of in a few paragraphs. The discussion of the complete problem has often been avoided by scientists because it is so exasperatingly complex. It is certainly not an easy problem for laymen when it is so tough for scientists.

We have listed the maintenance chemicals as item number 5 on our list of environmental requirements. Actually, item number 5 consists of approximately forty separate items each of which by itself constitutes a daily or at least consistent need. When the problem of the balance between all these items is contemplated, it seems like an insurmountable one. However, we shall not dodge it or fail to discuss the ways in which human beings can attempt to solve it. It is a practical problem involving forty variables which face everyone. It must be solved, perhaps in a helter-skelter way, by everyone who continues to remain alive. Fortunately nature helps us solve it, as we shall see in the next chapter; also fortunately we are so built that we can tolerate what may be regarded as far from the ideal proportions with respect to the different maintenance items.

The maintenance chemicals which, like oxygen and water, must be obtained from our environment daily are listed below along with a *rough* estimate of the daily amounts required.

Maintenance Chemicals*

Minerals† (mostly in ionic form)

Sodium (5 g), potassium (4 g), calcium (0.8 g), magnesium (0.35 g), phosphate (2 g), chloride (7 g), fluoride (0.5 mg), iodide (0.1 mg), manganese (5 mg), zinc (15 mg), iron (15 mg), copper (2 mg), chromium (2 mg), molybdenum (0.5 mg), cobalt, (0.1 mg), selenium (0.5 mg).

Amino Acids‡

Valine (0.6 g), threonine (0.3 g), leucine (0.8 g), lysine (1.6 g), isoleucine (0.5 g), phenylalanine (0.8 g), methionine (2 g), trytophan (0.15 g).

Vitamins, etc.§

Vitamin A (alcohol) (1.5 mg), vitamin C (ascorbic acid) (45 mg), vitamin D (calciferol) (0.01 mg), vitamin E (alpha tocopherol) (15 mg), vitamin K (2 mg), thiamin (1.2 mg), riboflavin (1.5 mg), pantothenic acid (10 mg), niacinamide (15 mg), pyridoxin (2 mg), folic acid (0.4 mg), biotin (0.2 mg), cobalamine (0.003 mg), choline (1 g), linoleic acid (10 g).

*In a different category from these maintenance chemicals is inert roughage or fiber which is nutritionally valuable because it gives the intestinal tract bulk which is mechanically desirable. An estimated 25 g of bulk, mostly cellulose, is consumed daily.
†The list of minerals and the approximate amounts of each required daily demands some explanation. In the first place the list is itself not a final or absolutely certain one. It is possible that other elements such as tin, vanadium, boron and possibly others should be added to the list. Some nutritionists would exclude from the list elements like chromium and selenium for which the evidence is not clear cut. The *amounts* listed for several of the minerals are rough estimates based largely on the amounts obtained when we eat good food. This is true for the amounts of sodium, potassium, chloride, fluoride, manganese, copper, chromium, molybdenum, cobalt and selenium. The amounts listed for calcium, magnesium, phosphate, iodide, zinc and iron are rough averages derived from more extensive studies and agree approximately with the rec-

These approximately forty maintenance chemicals which must be supplied from our nutritional environment constitute the A, B, C's of modern nutrition, and no scientific approach to nutrition can be made without their consideration. If we are forced to do so, we can get adequate nutrition leaving out and forgetting about lettuce, tomatoes, beefsteak, beans or any other specific single food. We cannot, however, by any stretch get life-supporting nutrition by leaving out any one of the essential maintenance chemicals.

ommendations of the Food and Nutrition Board (*Recommended Dietary Allowances*, 8th ed. Washington, D.C., National Academy of Sciences [1974], publication 2216). It would be possible to enter into an extensive documented debate with respect to the requirements for every item on the entire list of maintenance chemicals including the minerals, but this is undesirable and out of place. We cannot, however, discuss these requirements intelligently unless we have some idea of the amounts involved.

A complicating factor in making these tabulations is the fact that how much one needs of one mineral is often greatly influenced by the supply of other minerals. All requirements listed are very approximate.

‡This list of nutritionally essential amino acids is a well-recognized one, and the requirements as listed are rough averages. These are based on determinations on a limited number of adults. An adult will gradually lose the nitrogen from his or her body unless the requirement for each and every essential amino acid is met daily. The ranges of daily needs in milligrams for individual adults in the original studies are as follows: Valine, 375 to 800; threonine, 103 to 500; leucine, 170 to 1100; lysine, 400 to 2800; isoleucine, 250 to 700; phenylalanine, 420 to 1100; methionine, 800 to 3000; tryptophan, 82 to 250. (See Amino acid requirements in index.)

We shall later discuss the fact that the list of essential amino acids is not as hard and fast as it might be and that amino acids other than those listed are nutritionally desirable and may be essential under some circumstances. The tabulation of the amounts of the essential amino acids required is made more difficult because, for example, the need for phenylalanine is decreased if tyrosine is supplied, the need for methionine is decreased if cystine is supplied, and the need for tryptophane hinges in part on how much niacinamide is in the diet.

§The items listed under this heading and their supposed daily requirements are subject to many qualifications and reservations which we will not discuss in detail here. The estimates for the first thirteen items are roughly in agreement with the recommendations of the Food and Nutrition Board (*Recommended Dietary Allowances,* 8th ed. Washington, D.C., National Academy of Sciences [1974], publication 2216). Of these requirements, those for vitamin A and vitamin C are seriously misleading as will be clear from later discussions. Choline and linoleic acid are not vitamins in the usual sense but they are nonetheless important nutritionally. The *amounts* listed are rough estimates based on what we get when we consume wholesome food. Almost every quantitative estimate in the entire list of maintenance chemicals is subject to some modification based on the relative availability of other nutrients or of other environmental conditions. To take an extreme case, the need for vitamin D is determined in part by the available sunshine. When the right amount of sunshine prevails nutritional vitamin D can be dispensed with entirely.

CHAPTER 2

HOW WE ARE ABLE TO GET THE NUTRIENTS WE NEED

NEITHER HUMAN BEINGS nor other earthly organisms could live were it not for the underlying biochemical unity in nature. All organisms are metabolically closely related and are completely interdependent so far as their nutrition is concerned.

This chemical unity is illustrated by the fact that with possibly a few exceptions every maintenance chemical listed in the previous chapter is common to and is a necessary part of the metabolic machinery of every kind of living thing. A substantial number of other biochemicals which we do not have to get from our environment is also found in all living machinery.

Because of this fact, when we consume the tissues of plants or animals we are likely to get *some kind of an assortment* of the maintenance chemicals we require. The only way one could be sure of getting a diet free from zinc, molybdenum, tryptophan, methionine, thiamin, pyridoxin or almost any other item on the list would be to avoid consuming the tissues of plants or animals. One's diet would be restricted to pure sugar, corn syrup (glucose), starch and refined fat. The moment we include plant or animal tissues in our diet, we are likely to get *some* of everything we need.

The quantitative aspects of nutrition, however, are crucially important. If one were to consume in one day one gram of each of the maintenance chemicals listed in the previous chapter, he would die before sunset because of the poisonous effects at this level of copper, molybdenum, fluoride, cobalt, iodide, selenium and perhaps other items on the list.

If one were to go to the other extreme and consume, in addition to energy sources, only one milligram of each of the maintenance chemicals each day for a period of time, he would not die promptly, but he would lose protein, minerals and vitamins from his body and would sooner or later become debilitated and helpless. He would be getting enough of some of the nutrients, but would be obtaining insignificant amounts of some of the others.

We are protected from the most flagrant imbalances when we consume the tissues of plants or animals because the make-ups of the metabolic machinery of different species show strong resemblances. Certain elements, for example, are not only relatively rare in nature but are present in metabolic machinery in very small but indispensable amounts. These are often called "trace elements," and in general the same ones are found in trace amounts in all plant, animal or bacterial tissues. The elements which are present in larger amounts in our bodies, such as phosphorus (phosphates), potassium, calcium and magnesium, tend to be present in relatively large amounts in all kinds of plant and animal tissues. Nature thus protects us from getting in our food massive amounts of what should be "trace" elements (these would kill us) and trifling amounts of the elements we need in larger amounts.

While there is certainly no general rule to cover all cases, there is a tendency for plant and animal tissues to be at least grossly "in balance" rather than "out of balance" so far as the various types of nutrients are concerned. In other words, we are not likely when eating plant and animal tissues to get enormous amounts of any nutrient which is needed in trace amounts, nor will we get miniscule amounts of nutrients which are needed in relatively large amounts.

The entire environmental picture, however, is painted with the same broad brush. We never expect to find the perfect climatic environment where the temperature day and night, summer and winter, is always just right, and where the humidity, rainfall, sunshine and wind are all tempered to please us. Likewise, we never should expect to find the perfect food environment, the perfect food growing on trees that bear the year around.

With respect to our entire environment, we must therefore be discriminatingly selective and aggressive in striving to modify our environment and adapt ourselves as best we can to the conditions which nature provides.

Furthermore, this striving, adaptation and selection must be continuous on a day-to-day or even an hour-to-hour basis. We cannot say, "Such and such clothing is suitable and we will wear it." Later in the day or in the month the clothing we have chosen may be entirely unsuitable. Similarly, we cannot establish a policy and say to ourselves, "We will eat cheese and crackers." While on occasion this food may seem suitable, at a later time it may be unavailable or seem quite inappropriate.

Life as a whole is a complicated process; it consists largely of being discriminating and selective in modifying and adapting to the environment which surrounds us: the climate, weather, food, the social and cultural milieu in which we find ourselves.

It becomes obvious that the adaptation to our food environment is very far from simple, especially if we seek to have the best. It is easy enough by simple diversification to get some kind of an assortment of the maintenance items we require. But if these needs are at all exacting (this will be discussed in later chapters), the achievement of something approaching optimal nutrition may be a far more taxing process than we imagine and may require far more expertise than most of us possess.

Human beings and all other organisms are in the same boat in the sense that they never encounter in nature a perfect food environment. It is easy to calculate that yeast cells in an ordinary small cake of compressed yeast will, if given excellent nutrition for one week, produce in that time over a billion tons of yeast. Yeast cells never encounter this kind of nutrition in nature. Fruit juice, for example, is far from an optimal culture medium for yeast. Corn growing in a field may produce all the way from 0 to 200 bushels per acre depending on the suitability of the environment. Never does it grow under such conditions that the temperature, sunlight, water supply, carbon dioxide supply, oxygen supply to the roots, and all the minerals (including trace minerals and nitrogen sources) are perfectly adjusted for optimal development.

My first nutritional experiment was done, unwittingly, when I was a youngster about twelve years old. I had the bright idea of buying some baby chicks from a hatchery at five cents apiece and raising them in a few weeks to be broilers which I could sell at about forty cents each. This seemed like a sure shot to bring me a good profit, but it didn't work out. I knew nothing about chick nutrition, and on the grain diet I fed them they promptly began to die off, and the whole project was a failure. Now I know, a little too late, that chick nutrition is an exacting matter, and that if one wants to raise broilers, one has to study their nutritional needs carefully and take advantage of all modern knowledge in this field.

My first allegedly scientific nutritional experiment was done with baby rats about fifteen years later. This time I fed the rats a grain and seed mixture which the animal dealer sold me, and I watched their development for a week. The baby rats gained on an average of something over a gram a day apiece. Their rate of development was doubled, however, when I changed their diet to one containing a substantial amount of casein. Evidently the grain and seed mixture which the animal dealer bragged about as being "just the thing" for them was far from optimal, especially in the light of the fact that we now know how to feed baby rats so they will grow and develop (their bodies grow and develop in every respect without becoming obese) and gain at the rate of five to seven grams per day.

Rats in nature are probably lucky if they live where they can get a good supply of grain of most any sort. On this they will live and propagate. However, this is far from an optimal diet; they get some kind of an assortment of the maintenance chemicals they require, but if they can get some cheese (casein) or its equivalent, they do much better. Never are they fed in nature as well as they are in an up-to-date nutritional laboratory.

"Surely," I tell myself, "it is evident to you that the principle of the imperfect environment which applies to all other kinds of organisms also applies to the species to which you belong—*homo sapiens*." A little reflection will convince us that the vast majority of human beings live with nutrition which is far from optimal and that hundreds of millions of children are developing below their potential because their nutritional environment is of poor or mediocre quality. Surely our nutritional environments are universally subject to improvement in the same sense as are the nutritional environments of yeast cells, corn plants and baby chicks or rats.

My own background makes this very real to me because throughout a lengthy scientific career I have been engaged in learning how to improve the nutritional environment of various kinds of organisms.

It was while I was learning how to improve the nutritional environment of yeast cells that I discovered, more than forty years ago, the existence of what I called "pantothenic acid," (meaning in Greek "from everywhere"). It was found in every kind of living cell tested. When this was isolated and identified and became available in pure form, it became evident that when used intelligently, the substance could not only improve the nutritional environment of yeast cells but also of many plants and all fowls and mammals. All organisms must have coenzyme A in their make-up, and pantothenic acid is an essential building stone for it.

At the time pantothenic acid was discovered and given its name, it was vaguely supposed that this substance was unique in having such a widespread distribution in all living things. Now we know better. The maintenance chemicals we have listed in the previous chapter as essential in our nutrition are, for the most part, ubiquitous, and are found in every kind of living thing.

These maintenance chemicals are never found ready-packaged in ideal proportions for us or for any other organism. Living with our nutritional environment and adapting to it is an exacting task worthy of our serious attention. Indeed, we can get from our environment the maintenance chemicals we need, but in line with nature's plan we must strive and use our intelligence if we are to get a really good assortment for ourselves and our children.

CHAPTER 3

MAJOR HISTORICAL BOUTS WITH THE FOOD ENVIRONMENT

COUNTLESS RECORDED and unrecorded famines have resulted from the inability of the human race to cope with the food-environment problem. In this discussion we will not, however, be concerned with these; rather we will deal with the large-scale problems which had their roots in the poor *quality* of the food consumed.

One of the fundamental difficulties which arises in connection with the food-environment problem is that food is not always eaten the moment it is procured. In this case there must be some means of keeping or storing the food before it is consumed. In primitive cultures, especially perhaps in arid regions, drying has been a prominent means of food preservation. Fruits, meats and fish have all been dried on a large scale for human consumption. Primitive drying involves, of course, more than mere drying. It usually involves exposure to sun and to the oxygen of the air, in addition. The exposure to air tends to destroy one of our essential nutrients, ascorbic acid, and for this reason food dried in a primitive way always has its nutritional value impaired.

For human beings the destruction of ascorbic acid in the drying process is of unusual importance because of our peculiar relationship to this substance. We need this substance at every stage of our existence, and the only source is the food we eat. Many other mammals—cattle, sheep, horses, dogs, cats and rats—need it just as badly as we do, but they have by inheritance the internal machinery for making ascorbic acid from available carbohydrates. This production takes place within their bodies continuously and is essential to their well-being. For cattle and horses dried hay is substantially as nutritious as the grass from which it is derived;

12

the fact that it has lost its ascorbic acid in the drying process does not impair its food value for the animals that make it endogenously.

For guinea pigs, however, the situation is different; they live and thrive on green leaves and grasses but dried hay cannot support them. They are among the few species (which include man) which need exogenous ascorbic acid continuously and must get it directly from their food. This is true also of our relatives the primates.

It is interesting that some types of organisms, including many bacteria and higher forms such as insects, have little or no need for ascorbic acid at any time. It is also true that green plants appear to produce and use it, but it does not appear to be universally needed by all cells. Seeds in general contain none or very little. When they sprout, it begins to appear, and in green leaves it is often relatively abundant and is doubtless physiologically and biochemically functional and essential.

In extreme cases human beings or animals which need exogenous ascorbic acid and are deprived of it contract scurvy which appears with varying degrees of severity. This disease was probably first observed about 1260 A.D. It was common in the British Navy until a surgeon, James Lind, recognized its dietary origin about 1750 and began giving seamen citrus fruit which served as a preventative. The nickname "Limeys" was given to British seamen because of this fact.

Overt scurvy appeared predominantly when people were forced to subsist on dried, as opposed to fresh, food. It occurred in armies and in sailors on long sea voyages. Statistics indicate that during the Crimean War (1853 to 1856) 26,000 cases of scurvy appeared among the French troops alone. During the American Civil War it has been estimated that 15 percent of the deaths were from scurvy.

In spite of the fact that ascorbic acid was one of the first vitamins to be discovered, there are still many simple questions regarding it which are unanswered. One of the simple unanswered questions is. "How much do we need for optimal health?"

Up until recent years the tendency has been to think that our needs are fulfilled if overt scurvy is prevented, but this concept is now seriously questioned. It has been estimated that young guinea pigs need over 100 times as much ascorbic acid for maximum development and for best wound healing when they are injured as is required to prevent the common scurvy symptoms.[1,2]

Some human experiments which may not yet be sufficiently well-conducted or clear-cut to convince everyone point to the conclusion that ascorbic acid needs are far greater than they have appeared to be.[3,4,5] Some scientists and some physicians are convinced that human beings benefit from one gram or more of ascorbic acid daily. This is in sharp contrast to the "recommended dietary allowance" of the Food and Nutrition Board of 45 mg. per day.[6] The answer to the question, "How much ascorbic acid does one need?" is a highly important one from the standpoint of public health and needs to be settled by careful investigation. If indeed it is true that human beings benefit from far larger amounts of ascorbic acid, then many millions are failing to gain optimal health for this reason.

Another unanswered question about ascorbic acid is, "What does it do for us physiologically and biochemically?" It has long been known that ascorbic acid is an antioxidant and probably this is part of its role. There is a strong suspicion, however, that ascorbic acid has other functions related to various enzyme systems. It is now known that the hydroxyl group in hydroxyproline and hydroxylysine cannot be incorporated physiologically without its presence. Collagen building depends on these hydroxy acids and cannot take place without the participation of ascorbic acid. Since collagen is the most abundant protein in the body and plays a supportive role throughout our body tissues, the role of ascorbic acid is a vital one. Its entire functioning is, however, shrouded in a fog of ignorance. There are strong reasons for thinking that the complex problem of immunity involves ascorbic acid in a crucial way, but this requires further exploration.

Another historical bout with the food-environment problem was ushered in with the milling of rice, a grain which has served dominantly as a most important human food.

Milled rice is not only more attractive in appearance, but it keeps incomparably better, especially in tropical, humid climates. It therefore became a staple food for millions in the Orient, and out of its too exclusive use arose the disease beriberi. Eijkman, a Dutch physician, discovered in 1897 that fowls fed a diet of polished rice contracted polyneuritis, which is closely related to the human disease beriberi.

When rice is milled, the product, polished rice, has the outer layers and most of the germ removed. It still has in it some of all the nutrients we need, but the thiamin (vitamin B_1) level is very low and its deficiency becomes the dominant one. It is interesting that the vitamin B_1 level in polished rice is just about right for the production of polyneuritis in fowls. The polished rice contains enough vitamin B_1 to keep fowls alive long enough to exhibit the disease. If fowls are fed a diet completely free from vitamin B_1 they simply die promptly without ever exhibiting the symptoms of polyneuritis.

The human death toll from beriberi over many decades must have been enormous. Of course, no reliable statistics are available because the nature of the disease remained unknown, and no doctors were available in the most afflicted regions to diagnose the disease. As late as 1925 in Japan alone, there were estimated to be 15,000 deaths per year from beriberi.[7]

The death toll alone gives an inadequate idea of the prevalence of and importance of the malnutrition incident to the use of polished rice as nearly the sole article of diet. For every person who died of the disease there were probably at least a score whose health was impaired to a lesser degree. The number of children and young people who failed to develop to their full potential because of a dominantly white rice diet must have been enormous.

The history of beriberi and the incidence of the consumption of polished rice lends support to the statement made in an earlier chapter that a large part of the human race lives and has lived under nutritional conditions which are far from optimal. Even now beriberi is far from eradicated.[8]

The hard facts of human history tell us that, practically speaking, polished rice is a remarkable food. It can be consumed at very high levels and with minimum supplementation and is still able to sustain human life. We have found in our laboratories that rice seems to have this ability also with experimental animals. My own interpretation, however, is that the life so sustained is liable to be at a very low level of quality. People who live largely on polished rice and barely escape beriberi are often as poorly nourished as is corn growing in a field and producing two to five bushels per acre. No one can say that the corn, under these conditions, is not alive.

My basis for this interpretation is the well-known fact, based on animal experimentation, that polished rice has low nutritional value in several respects. Even with vitamin B₁ added, it constitutes a poor diet. It not only is conspicuously deficient in certain minerals and amino acids but also in a number of vitamins other than vitamin B₁. Polished rice can be enormously and successfully improved for animals if appropriate minerals, amino acids and vitamins are added to it. On this point, with respect to animals, there can be no question whatever. To me it seems obvious that similar levels of improvement could be instituted if we were to experiment with human beings.

Along with my interpretation goes the belief that if the milling of rice had never been instituted and if people had found some way to keep brown rice and use it as almost a sole article of diet, malnutrition would not have been avoided. It is true that beriberi would never have occurred, but the people who consumed an exclusive brown rice diet would still have been impaired because of poor nutrition. Their level of nutrition in case brown rice were used would have been raised so that perhaps it would be comparable to that of corn growing in a field and producing ten to fifteen bushels per acre instead of the 200 bushels or more that is possible. Experimental animals on a brown rice diet thrive better than on polished rice, but even so their nutrition is a far cry from that which can be provided by expert attention to all the detailed nutritional needs.

Another historical bout with the food-environment problem came about primarily because of the too exclusive use in human dietaries of another grain—corn. This happened in Spain, Italy, Egypt and in the southern states of the United States. In the United States there were at one stage about 170,000 cases of pellagra and 20,000 deaths from this disease each year. As a result of the work of Dr. Joseph Goldberger and others, overt pellagra has now practically disappeared from the southern United States.

While corn is an excellent food for fattening grown cattle, it is nutritionally inferior to rice or wheat for humans. As ruminants, cattle have rumen microorganisms working for them to make possible their subsistence on food which otherwise could not sustain life. (The nutrition of calves is much more exacting, and whole corn does not suffice for them.)

For human beings whole corn is relatively deficient in two related nutrients—tryptophan, which can be converted in the body to niacinamide, and niacinamide itself. These and nearly all other necessary nutrients are present in corn, but their levels are too low for a reasonably balanced human food. Whole corn as a sole article of diet is extremely deficient for babies and growing children.

Even primitive people, presumably based upon long human experience, have a tendency to watch the nutrition of babies and children more than that of adults. Hence, even where poverty induces the adults to live largely on cornbread and sow belly, the babies and children tend to get somewhat better nutrition. If they had not, they would not have survived.

Rickets is an environmental disease which has a more complex origin than scurvy, beriberi or pellagra.[9] The nature and origin of this disease, which of course involves poor bone development, has been elucidated by animal experimentation since rickets can be induced in many animals, including fowls, under conditions similar to those which produce the disease in children.

There are three distinct nutrients involved in producing rickets: calcium, phosphate and vitamin D. If any one of these three nutritional items is lacking in the diet or is seriously out of balance, rickets results.

Vitamin D is a unique nutrient in that it can be dispensed with entirely provided adequate but not excessive levels of ultraviolet light are available. In this case vitamin D is produced in the skin on exposure to sunlight, and it ceases to be a necessary nutrient. Because vitamin D can be produced endogenously, some would prefer to think of it as a hormone. Like the thyroid hormone, it can be consumed or produced endogenously. In order for the thyroid hormone to be produced endogenously, a special nutrient, iodine, is needed. No special nutrient is required for endogenous vitamin D production.

Historically, rickets has been most common in cities during the winter in the temperate zone. Under these conditions, children did not get enough sunlight, and if their diets were deficient or poorly balanced with respect to calcium and phosphate, this poor balance was a contributing factor. Codliver oil was given to children for centuries before it was known to be a good source of vitamin D and A. When codliver oil was used, it served as an environmental substitute for sunshine.

Kwashiorkor is the name given to a childhood disease of malnutrition which has been found dominantly in underdeveloped countries.[10] This disease, which causes severe physical and mental retardation, is often thought of as due primarily to protein (amino acid) deficiency. The diets of children who contract this disease are, however, deficient in many ways. While poor amino acid nutrition alone could be responsible, it has been found in our laboratories that the common food "proteins" usually carry with them (unless exhaustively purified) a considerable assortment of B vitamins, and it is likely that kwashiorkor results from multiple deficiencies in addition to amino acid deficiencies.

In all of these historical bouts with the food-environment which have resulted in disease there is a common element which needs to be noted and discussed in more detail in a later chapter. This is the matter of susceptibility. When a crew of sailors all ate the same food, certain individuals became severely afflicted with scurvy while others escaped. When a population eats polished rice exclusively, not all contract beriberi, only certain individuals. If we are to be realistic, we must consider these and other similar facts and seek to understand them. This problem will be discussed later.

We have sought in this brief chapter not to discuss all the difficulties which may arise because of failure to cope with the nutritional environment. We have noted only some of the outstanding examples where poor (and ignorant) handling of the nutritional environment has resulted in overt and well-recognized diseases.

REFERENCES

1. Williams, R.J., and Deason, G.: Individuality in vitamin C needs. *Proc. Natl. Acad. Sci. USA*, 57:1638, 1967.
2. Yew, Man-Li S.: Recommended daily allowance of vitamin C. *Proc. Natl. Acad. Sci. USA*, 70:963, 1973.

3. Anderson, T.W., Reid, D.W., and Barton, G.H.: Vitamin C and the common cold: A double-blind trial. *Can. Med. Assoc. J.*, *107*:503, 1972.
4. Wilson, C.M., and Loh, H.S.: Common cold and vitamin C. *Lancet*, *1*:638, 1973.
5. Coulson, J.L., et al.: Vitamin C prophylaxis in a boarding school. *N. Engl. J. Med.*, *290*:6, 1974.
6. Food and Nutrition Board: *Recommended Dietary Allowances*, 8th ed. Washington, D.C., Natl. Acad. Sci., 1974, publication 2216.
7. Williams, R.R.: *Toward the Conquest of Beriberi.* Cambridge, Harvard U Pr, 1961.
8. Goldberger, J.: In Terris, M. (Ed): *Goldberger on Pellagra*, Baton Rouge, La. State U Pr, 1969.
9. Hess, A.F.: *Rickets.* Philadelphia, Lea & Febiger, 1929.
10. De Silva, C.C., and Baptist, N.G.: *Tropical Nutritional Disorders of Infants and Children.* Springfield, Thomas, 1969.

CHAPTER 4

WHAT ARE THE BASIC PRINCIPLES WHICH UNDERLIE NUTRITIONAL SCIENCE?

NUTRITIONAL SCIENCE with all its ramifications and implications is grossly underdeveloped. Its basic principles have heretofore not been set forth, and this we will attempt to do.

1. *All organisms utilize continuously their own metabolically derived energy.* This energy, the use of which is essential to and intimately intertwined with all life activities, has its ultimate origin in the sun, but is made available by reason of special biochemical transformations which living organisms are able to perform. In mammals and many other organisms the dominant process for getting this internal energy is a complicated burning of fuel substances which must be obtained from the environment. This burning is brought about through the agency of many enzyme catalysts.

2. *The catabolism (burning) of suitable types of fuel by mammals not only provides indispensable energy but also yields essential intermediates for the biosynthesis of those cellular components which can be produced endogenously. Poorly balanced fuel mixtures can cause the accumulation of intermediates which can be detrimental.* Too much use of amino acids, fat acids and alcohol for energy purposes can cause difficulties (sometimes serious) for known and unknown reasons. Growing evidence indicates that some carbohydrates, notably sucrose (see sugar consumption), may also be damaging when used excessively as an energy source.

3. *All organisms, to make it possible for them to derive energy and carry out essential functions, require from their environment many nonfuel nutrients (raw materials) for building and maintain-*

ing their operating metabolic machinery. This intricate machinery built from many raw materials, or building blocks, makes possible the burning of fuel, the release of energy, and the metabolism which is the basis of all living activities. For mammals, the environmentally derived building blocks for the construction of basic metabolic machinery are dominantly minerals, amino acids and the B vitamins.

4. *Mammals, representing multicellular organisms, require other nonfuel nutrients not known to be used directly in the building of the basic metabolic machinery common to all living cells.* This somewhat indefinite group of nutrients includes vitamin A, ascorbic acid, vitamin D, vitamin E, vitamin K, and probably others. Vitamin A acid which can replace vitamin A in all its functions, except those involving the production of visual pigments, may also belong in this group, but how it functions is so obscure that it is impossible to classify it. If it, or any other nutrient, is needed by all cells, it does not belong in this group.

These nutrients, as a group, are needed for highly specialized purposes, such as building visual machinery, and for other purposes (presently obscure) probably associated with cell, tissue and organ coordination in complex mammalian systems. Hormone production may be one of the associated functions.

5. *The cell is the unit of life; it is also the center of all metabolic activity, and the unit which must be adequately nourished.* The nourishment of a complex multicellular organism like a mammal cannot be studied merely as a wholesale operation. *All* the cells in the entire organism must be considered from the standpoint of the adequacy or inadequacy of their nourishment. The important applicability of this principle will become more evident from the discussion in Chapters 5 and 8.

6. *The metabolic machinery in all living cells has common characteristics and is built from many of the same structural units.* The very same chemical entities—certain minerals, trace minerals, amino acids, purine and pyrimidine bases, ribose and deoxyribose, fat acids, choline, many vitamins, etc.—are found universally in the cellular metabolic machinery of plant and animal organisms irrespective of their phylum, class, order, family, genus or species. These fundamental structural units must, in the case of each unit and each cell,

be either furnished in the food or built up endogenously by the cell from available raw materials. The metabolic machinery in human cells is in its essentials and with respect to its structural units very similar to what is present in yeast cells, bacteria, insects, green plants, fowls and fishes.

7. *By nature and inheritance, different organisms and different cells show wide variance in their ability to build the organic chemical structures needed for the construction of metabolic machinery.* Some are able to produce many of the necessary structural units readily, in which case these units are not needed nutritionally. Other organisms must get many of these same units from the environment. Differing synthetic abilities, rather than differences in the structural units involved, accounts largely for the differing nutritional needs of diverse organisms. The mineral needs of different organisms are very similar; there is no transmutation or building of needed elements.

8. *Organisms throughout the entire biological kingdom are nutritionally completely dependent on each other.* For example, it is extremely common in nature, if not universal, for organisms to derive many of the structural units needed for building metabolic machinery from other organisms, and to be completely dependent on these sources of supply. Life on earth could not continue if disunity existed, if every kind of organism had its own unique structural units from which its metabolic machinery had to be built. These building *units* are not merely *similar*; they are *identical*.

The phenomena of nutritional interdependence can be observed to a degree among the cells in a mammalian body. For example, glutamine is not an "essential" amino acid for the human body as a whole, but is essential for certain cells. This means that it is produced by some other cells and thus furnished to those that need it. There are quite possibly many cases of this sort hitherto unrecognized. Such observations may be important because under some circumstances (impairment of the cells which commonly produce it) glutamine, for example, may become an amino acid which is nutritionally essential for good health.

9. *Organisms and cells do not find in nature ready-made, perfectly adjusted optimal assortments of nutrients; they commonly have to put up with imperfect nutrition.* This principle, from the

standpoint of day-to-day practicality, is one of the most important. It applies to all organisms—plant, animal, bacterial. Human beings, for example, are faced with the continuous necessity of searching, selecting, procuring, cultivating, preparing, shipping and storing food; and even with industry and the best of intentions they may not be able to come up with anything approaching perfect nutrition. An optimal food environment is as rare as a climatic environment where the temperature, humidity, wind, rainfall and sunshine are always just right. Practically speaking, nutrition is always subject to improvement.

Consideration of this principle leads us to wonder whether nutritional needs are not sometimes relative rather than absolute. For example, there is no question that certain amino acids are nutritionally essential for mammals, including human beings. Long ago it was observed, however, that while young rats could live without an exogenous source of arginine, they thrived better if it was furnished. It has also been found that animals are better nourished if they get a complete assortment of amino acids than if they get only the "essential" ones.

It is probable that nutrition can often be improved not only by providing a better assortment of essential nutrients but also by providing desirable "nonessentials." The hard and fast concept that amino acids (or other nutrients) are always either absolutely "essenitl" or else absolutely "nonessential" is probably fallacious.

Nutritional requirements from the quantitative standpoint are often complex. The need for certain important items can be greatly influenced by the availability of other nutrients. For example, the need for choline hinges on the availability of methionine. Methionine needs are lessened when cystine is abundantly supplied; phenylalanine needs are decreased if tyrosine is supplied; niacinamide can be dispensed with if sufficient trytophan is furnished. Considerations such as these need to be thought of in connection with principles 10, 11 and 12 stated below.

10. *The various nonfuel nutrients whatever they may be and wherever they may be effective always work together as a team to make metabolism and life activities possible.* For example, the large array of structural units needed to build metabolic machinery is like a series of nuts, bolts, wheels, spindles, gears, cams, chains and belts,

etc. which enter into the make-up of a complicated machine. Single nutrients as such are effective only when they participate in teamwork. A failure to recognize this principle has led to the fallacy of looking at vitamins and other nutrients as *drugs* or *medicines*, which they are not. Drugs which are typically foreign to the body do not participate constructively; by themselves they may interfere with metabolic operations, hopefully in an overall beneficial way and with a minimum of undesired effects.

We cannot hope to understand the essentials of human nutrition if we think of nutrients as "magic bullets" which by themselves are expected to perform miracles. There is an old German saying, "Ohne Phosphor, keine Gedanken." This is true but completely misleading. Phosphorus or more properly phosphate is a vital component of metabolic machinery, and no process associated with life can take place without it. But there are dozens of other components of metabolic machinery for which this is also true. It cannot be emphasized too strongly that phosphate and all other nutrients always act as members of a team. We can truthfully say, "without zinc we cannot think," but this merely means that zinc is a member of the metabolic team.

11. *The essential and vital nutritional teamwork can be impeded or impaired* (a) *by a deficient supply of any nutrient,* (b) *by the presence of numerous agents which may interfere in many ways,* (c) *by the excess concentration of normal metabolites,* (d) *by imbalances with respect to the team members,* (e) *by emotional or other stress.* The deleterious *agents* referred to above include poisons, drugs, natural toxicants in foods (see Ch. 10), and allergens which characteristically only affect biochemically vulnerable individuals. The various enemies of good nutrition need extensive study from the standpoint of fundamental, detailed metabolism because our knowledge of many of them is scanty. Problems related to the enemies of nutrition will be discussed in later chapters.

12. *By inheritance, each member of the human family is a unique specimen with respect to his or her pattern of metabolic activities and the quantitative aspects of his or her nutritional requirements* (see Ch. 7). This principle is much broader inasmuch as it also applies to other organisms including animals. Hence, this individuality can be studied in the laboratory.

The importance of this principle becomes apparent when it is recognized that the differences between individuals are often far from trifling (Ch. 7), and that the only kind of people who need or can use nutrition are *individual* people.

The twelve principles we have stated above are not presented with any degree of finality. It seems that the principles, whatever they are, need badly to be stated and pondered. At least half of the twelve proposed principles have novel features not hitherto considered. All of these principles are based, we believe, on biological facts, not theories, and it seems that their recognition will have the effect of directing nutritional research into many new and promising channels.

If underlying principles are neglected, nutritional science must remain sickly. It tends to become a jumble of unrelated observations, facts and figures often relatively meaningless and realistically inapplicable. Nutritional science cannot develop piecemeal in a biological vacuum.

The whole problem of food—its selection, cultivation, preparation, processing, storage, buying and selling—is of major concern to all of humanity. The benefits of agriculture, food technology and the supermarket depend absolutely upon nutritional value, and the benefits can be lost if we do not have a well-ordered, biologically oriented nutritional science to help us judge, conserve and utilize nutritional values. Whatever other attractive features foods may have, they are worthless as foods unless they contribute nutritional value. If we continue to give intelligence in this area a low priority (as we do in all our schools), this is unwittingly taking the ridiculous position that quality in foods is of no concern.

In succeeding chapters we will have occasions to allude to and discuss in more detail some of the basic principles set forth briefly above. If we have oversimplified them, it has been done in order to stress certain vital considerations which have hitherto been neglected.

CHAPTER 5

INTERNAL NUTRITION

AN UNCRITICAL VIEW might lead one to say, "If one reveals what is eaten for breakfast, lunch, dinner and between times, it will be evident what the quality of his nutrition is."

There are two important and rather obvious *assumptions* underlying such a statement. One is that food that is eaten is always digested; the second is that food which is digested is subsequently absorbed readily and ultimately delivered to points where it is needed.

In a thoroughgoing realistic nutritional science, we need to be concerned not just with what food we put into our mouths but, more importantly, with the fuel substances, maintenance chemicals, etc., which get to the cells and tissues of our bodies where all the metabolic activities are going on.

Fundamentally, the metabolically active cells in our body are what need nourishment, and a vital question is whether a good assortment of minerals, amino acids, and vitamins that these cells need is well supplied. The lettuce, tomatoes, beefsteak and beans that one may eat contribute only indirectly and remotely to cellular nutrition. They furnish to the digestive tract mostly in combined forms the chemical units the cells need. In nutritional science we must think of the steps intermediate between consuming food and nourishing the vital cells where all metabolism occurs.

Nutritionists have sometimes been guilty of thinking of digestion as an automatic process which proceeds willy nilly with approximate perfection. Carbohydrates are said to be digested best, about 98 percent, fats about 95 percent, and protein about 92 percent.

In a later chapter we will present information which tells us, realistically speaking, that such estimates are spurious when applied to real people.

How well digestion proceeds depends on the functioning of the varying digestive juices of individual persons and upon the particular carbohydrate, fat or protein to be digested. We will present more on this subject later.

Absorption is, of course, not primarily a simple sieve action but involves in many cases complicated enzyme systems. Comparatively little is known of the facts regarding the frequency and extent of malabsorption as it occurs in individual people. It is certain, however, that the *if* of absorption is a real factor which has to be taken into account when we consider the problems of nutrition in a definitive and detailed way.

An important assumption we make when we think of nutrition as involving only the consumption of food is that once digested and absorbed the products are automatically delivered adequately to the cells that need them.

In the author's scientific background there is much that has made him very sensitive to this problem. I was certainly one of the first in my generation to center attention on cellular nutrition and to find ways and means of improving the biochemical environment of living cells. Because of long experience in this area, it seems very natural for me to ask, "Do the cells all over the body automatically receive in an effective fashion all of the nutritional elements that have been absorbed?"

Little is actually *known* about the answer to this question. Contemplation suggests, however, that the answer is not obvious, and that maybe one's circulatory system is not always fully effective.

A highly pertinent observation in this connection is that the pumping capacities of the hearts of healthy young men have been found to vary from 3.16 to 10.81 liters of blood per minute.[1] This is more than a three-fold range. This would suggest that with other things being equal the chances of effective blood distribution may be three times as good in some individuals as in others.

The problem of distribution becomes more pointed when localized circulation is given attention. To the author, the proper distribution of *everything* the blood carries to every cell and tissue of the body seems like a logistic undertaking of tremendous proportions. It resembles continuously furnishing an army of many trillions with everything that is needed. It would be remarkable, indeed, if all tissues were always fed with complete impartiality and adequacy. To me, it is utterly ridiculous to *assume* that in any individual the distribution system works with perfection or approximate perfection to serve all local needs.

Whether any particular part of the body is unusually prone to be malnourished because of inefficient circulation is not known. However, there are a number of facts which suggest that the brain cells are often malnourished simply because the circulatory system is inadequate to do the job.

First is an incontrovertible fact that the carotid arteries which carry blood to the brain vary several-fold in blood-carrying capacity.[2] Let us suppose, for example, that an individual who has a heart with low pumping capacity also has unusually small carotid arteries. Is it not reasonable to suppose that such a person's brain cells would suffer, relatively at least, from malnutrition?

An observation which strongly suggests that this is so is the fact that some individuals become senile prematurely, while there are others (presumably with good cerebral circulation) who, in spite of other troubles, retain their mental faculties until an advanced age.

Statistical studies of brain cell counts on brains of different ages (accidental deaths) have led to the estimate that on the average an adult human being loses 1,000 to 2,000 brain cells per hour.[3] The question naturally arises in my mind, "Why do these brain cells die off?" And a quick answer is, "Because environmental conditions, including the nutritional environment, have become inadequate." I have suggested this question and this answer to a number of experts who are in the best position to know, and no one has yet provided another answer, nor has anyone seriously questioned the fundamental soundness of my answer.

It seems very probable to me, though I recognize that this is a speculation, that those individuals who have hearts with low pumping capacities and/or small carotid arteries probably lose brain cells at a much higher than average rate, 5,000 cells per hour, and are prone to become prematurely senile. On the other hand, those who have excellent cerebral circulation tend to lose brain cells at far lower rates than the average.

It is interesting and suggestive in this connection that it has been observed that the brains of alcoholics are so disintegrated as to be useless for dissection by medical students.[4,5] Certainly it seems reasonable to suppose that alcoholics lose brain cells far more rapidly than the average, and that aside from toxicity this is associated with the very poor nutritional environment furnished by the consumption of alcohol to the exclusion of nourishing foods.

The possibility of impaired cellular nutrition by reason of poor circulation is one that needs to be considered *in addition* to the possibility that nutrition may be of poor quality simply because the food consumed carries a poor assortment of nutritional items. If the assortment of maintenance chemicals picked up by the blood is a poor one, circulation of the highest quality cannot correct the defect.

A well-recognized *enemy* of good circulation is atherosclerosis which, as is well-known, is not limited in its incidence to elderly people but is found in middle-aged and even in young people (mainly soldiers). We have elsewhere called attention to the probability that this condition is promoted by poor cellular nutrition.[6,7]

One of the *friends* of good internal nutrition and effective circulation is suitable exercise. Exercise helps build up and maintain an effective heart and probably benefits indirectly every cell and tissue in the body. Measures to build up the circulation, in cases of individuals who particularly need this kind of help, have probably been inadequately explored and exploited.

The author makes no pretense, of course, of being an expert in the field of pathology. Because of my prolonged attention to the problems of cellular nutrition and my full recognition that in all of nature all cells live at graded (and often low) levels of efficiency because of the varying environments that surround them, I see a vast field of cellular pathology which, to the best of my knowledge, has not been touched by professional pathologists.

In my view, cells and tissues all over our bodies are liable to be in a pathological state (to varying degrees) if the environment supplied them is inadequate in quality (furnishing a poor assortment of metabolic units) or is limited in quantity due to generalized or localized poor circulation.

The author recognizes, or I think I do, that a hundred different unfavorable things can happen to brain cells before they actually die, and that a multitude of brain malfunctions, aside from those of senility, can result from poor environmental conditions surrounding the functioning cells. Those who are followers of Freud will do well to remember that it was his dream that someday the chemistry of the brain would be better understood and brought under control.[8]

There are two diseased conditions related to brain cell function with which I have either had personal experience or have studied professionally.

Late in my seventies I experienced total macular degeneration in the retina of my left eye. Many consultations and examinations later, I have become convinced that the primary problem was inadequate circulation in the macular region which probably has existed from birth but not to a degree to cause serious trouble until it was accentuated by atherosclerosis. Pictures showing excellent peripheral circulation in my eyes bear out the interpretation that macular circulation may have been marginal even during my youth. My peripheral vision in my left eye is excellent, and the two facts appear related. About two years after I lost the macular vision in my left eye (this happened in a period of a few months), my right eye showed unmistakable signs of going along the same route. Nothing could apparently be done to improve the anatomy of the blood vessels, so I took heroic measures to try to improve the *quality* of the blood which reached my retinas by using various carefully chosen nutritional supplements. Whether the favorable results can be attributed to these efforts I cannot say, but more than three years after I first saw that the macular vision in my right eye began to be impaired, I can still read with suitable lenses, and there has been no substantial change during the past two and a half years.

This experience, of course, proves nothing, but it does tend to strengthen my interpretation that brain cells, including retinal cells, do not die off if they are supplied with a good environment.

Another related diseased condition has occupied my professional attention for at least twenty years. This is alcoholism. I have come to the conclusion on the basis of long study that the most probable root of the trouble is cellular impairment in the brain. When the brain cells, including those which are involved in regulating appetites, are given a poor nutritional environment, as well as an environment polluted with alcohol which may be at poisonous levels, they become impaired. The ultimate and crucial result is that the afflicted individual eventually loses all desire for food but has a perverted appetite for alcohol. There are of course many ramifications of the disease, as with other diseases, but in my judgment the basic principle is simple.[9, 10]

Pathologists of the future will be concerned with such cellular impairments as we have been considering, not only in the brain but also in other organs and tissues of the body.

If our discussion concerning impairment of brain cells has validity, there is no reason whatever to suppose that the cells and tissues in other organs should be excluded from similar consideration. Kidneys, livers, hearts, intestines, muscles, endocrine glands, etc., may, for all current pathologists know, be subject to impairment and disease for similar reasons. There is always the possibility that these organs and tissues may suffer either because the food consumed is inadequate or because the assortment of nutrient elements is inadequately delivered by the local circulation.

REFERENCES

1. Ring, G.C., et al.: Pumping capacity of hearts. *J. Appl. Physiology*, *5*:99, 1952.
2. Anson, B.J.: *Atlas of Human Anatomy*. Philadelphia, Saunders, 1950.
3. Brody, H.: Organization of the cerebral cortex III: A study of ageing in human cerebral cortex, *J. Comp. Neurol.*, *102*:511, 1955.
4. Moskow, H.A., Pennington, R.C., and Knisley, M.H.: Alcohol, sludge and hypoxic areas of the nervous system, liver and heart. *Microvasc. Res.*, *1*:174, 1968.
5. Courville, C.B.: *Effects of Alcohol on the Nervous System*. Los Angeles, San Lucas Press, 1966.
6. Williams, R.J.: Nutrition and ischemic heart disease. *Borden's Rev. Nutr. Res. 31*:No. 2, April-June, 1971.
7. Williams, R.J.: *Nutrition Against Disease*. New York, Pitman, 1971, Ch. 5.
8. Freud, S.: *An Outline of Psychoanalysis*. New York, Norton, 1949.
9. Williams, R.J.: *Alcoholism: The Nutritional Approach*. Austin, U of Tex Pr, 1959.
10. Williams, R.J.: *Nutrition Against Disease*. New York, Pitman, 1971, Ch. 11.

CHAPTER 6

PRENATAL NUTRITION

A DEVELOPING FETUS presents an example *par excellence* of internal nutrition. *Everything* the fetus needs must be supplied by way of the circulating blood of the prospective mother, and growth and development depend absolutely on the needs being fully provided.

It has long been known in animals which commonly give birth to litters of young that sometimes a fetus is unfavorably located in the uterus and as a result gets a poor blood supply and becomes the "runt" of the litter—smaller, weaker and less able to compete for food after birth. In such a case the nutrition furnished during fetal development may have been of good quality, but the *amount* furnished was insufficient to produce what is thought of as normal development.

Let us ask ourselves the question, "Is fetal development sometimes impaired and retarded because the *quality* of the nutrition furnished is poor?" It is impossible to answer this question definitively in the absence of controlled experimentation. Merely to state that poor or mediocre nutrition may cause impaired fetal development should not carry much weight unless it is backed by scientific evidence, even though it seems a commonsense deduction.

Human experiments of the kind that can be done with animals seem out of the question, but experimental animals are expendable, and a tremendous body of evidence shows that the same principles apply to all mammals.

After I had discovered and isolated pantothenic acid and had paved the way for its commercial production, the question was often asked, "Is pantothenic acid really a vitamin needed by animals, including mammals, as well as by developing yeast cells?"

One of the many experiments which clearly supported an affirmative answer to this question was done in France.[1] It involved giving young female rats six different levels of this supposed vitamin, breeding them, and keeping a careful record of their ability to bear healthy young. The experiment involved sixty-six female rats, and the score showed plainly that their ability to reproduce was conditioned by a suitable level of pantothenic acid in their diet.

The seventeen female rats receiving no pantothenic acid and the ten rats receiving only 10 mcg per day bore no young whatever. Conception takes place by such rats, but resorption follows, not fetal development. Rats receiving 20 to 25 mcg per day also conceived, and 58 percent of the fetuses were resorbed, but 19 percent were born deformed, and 24 percent appeared normal at birth. The percentage of normal young increased at successively higher levels of pantothenic acid intake as follows:

30 to 35 mcg per day—38 percent normal

40 to 45 mcg per day—72 percent normal

50 mcg per day—95.5 percent normal

It is unfortunate that the 50 mcg per day level was the highest used in this experiment, because it has been estimated that twice this amount (100 mcg per day) is required for maximum growth in young rats. Probably a pregnant female rat needs even more than this for best performance.

This experiment with pantothenic acid demonstrates with the utmost clarity that fetal development can be seriously impaired, even abolished, by poor quality nutrition.

Some of the most striking demonstrations suggesting that all individual nutrients are needed for fetal development have been made with deficiencies of the vitamin *folic acid*.[2] This vitamin was first found to be essential in the environment of the cells of certain lactic acid bacteria. It was first concentrated and given its name in our laboratories and was subsequently shown to be essential for the environment of mammalian and other animal cells, as well as cells of lactic acid bacteria.

That it is essential for fetal development can be readily demonstrated by supplementing otherwise good diets with graded levels during pregnancy and at various stages of gestation. Numerous studies along this line have been carried out. In some cases where mild deficiencies have been induced, as high as 95 percent of the young have been deformed. If folic acid is excluded from the diet entirely, no young are produced.

Fourteen kinds of skeletal malformations have been induced by folic acid deficiency in rats. In addition, many deformities in internal organs have been induced: those of the heart, blood vessels, endocrine glands and brain. Sometimes animals are even born without heads; sometimes the brains develop outside the skull, etc.

To center one's attention on what the deficiency of one or two vitamins will do to reproduction gives a distorted view of the reproductive process where *every known nutrient* (and unknown ones too if they exist) is actually involved. One of the earliest evidences that individual nutrients are essential for healthy fetal development appeared when it was found decades ago that healthy sows gave birth to eyeless pigs when their diets were deficient in vitamin A, but when the same sows were fed exactly the same diet with adequate vitamin A added, the newborn pigs were quite normal.[3]

Deficiencies of individual minerals and of the nutritionally essential amino acids can also play havoc with the reproductive process, as has been demonstrated in numerous studies. There seems to be no doubt that fetuses need for healthy development a well-rounded environment containing all the essential minerals, trace minerals, amino acids, and vitamins, etc., and that too low a level of any of these essentials can interfere seriously with reproduction.

Nutrition during the reproductive cycle is more exacting than at other times. It has been found repeatedly that adult animals can subsist on diets which will not promote reproduction. That diets must be better during reproduction has been widely established for dogs, cats, rats, mice, foxes, monkeys, chickens, turkeys, and even fish.[4]

It may be observed widely throughout nature that organisms during early stages of development need nutrients that later on can be produced endogenously or are needed only at low levels.

In the plant world, seedlings derive from the storage material in the seed or from the soil organisms nutrients such as amino acids and vitamins which have no beneficial effect when supplied later to more mature plants. When pantothenic acid was first concentrated, we found it to stimulate the growth of very young plants. At later stages of development when it is produced endogenously no effect could be demonstrated.

In the insect world we have already noted that honeybees and houseflies can subsist on practically pure sugar. This is very far from true, however, with respect to insects during earlier stages of metamorphosis. Insect larvae, for example, have very complex nutritional requirements, including many of the amino acids and vitamins required routinely by mammalian organisms.

Profound changes in larval development can be induced in insects by modifying their diets. Bee larvae that are fed "royal jelly" become queen bees which live for years and produce many thousands of progeny, whereas the same larvae fed the routine diet become infertile worker bees that commonly live only a few weeks. It was particularly interesting to the author that for many years the richest known natural source of pantothenic acid was "royal jelly." Subsequently it has been found that codfish ovaries are a richer source. These facts point to the important role pantothenic acid plays in reproduction.

In view of all these and other facts involving organisms other than mammals, it is not surprising that mammals during fetal development must be well supplied with all the essential nutrients and that deficiencies during fetal development can have devastating effects.

It is interesting in this connection that the study of rat nutrition commonly begins with weanling animals. These have not only developed *in utero* for three weeks but have suckled their mothers for a similar period. For obvious reasons the nutrition of newborn rats has received practically no attention. It is very dangerous, however, to assume that the complete story of nutrition can be told on the basis of results obtained with *weanling* rats.

That the nutrition of newborn rats would be very exacting is indicated by the fact that when we shift our attention to the chick, an animal which can be studied when it is ready to enter the world at an embryonic age of only three weeks, its nutrition is found to be far more exacting than that of weanling rats. It was not until a large number of B vitamins had been discovered by microbiological methods that chick nutrition could be systematically studied. About seventy years ago weanling rats were found able to live on semisynthetic diets. Baby chicks, on the other hand, when fed such diets died promptly. Many years later, semisynthetic diets, including newly discovered vitamins, could be produced that would support life and substantial growth in baby chicks.

It seems that in nature we find a universal rule—organisms in their earlier developmental stages have very exacting nutrition. The farther back we go to the original event of conception, the more exacting the nutrition appears to be. An environment which will support an adult organism may be totally inadequate to support the life and development of an embryo or a very young specimen.

In the case of human beings (and other mammals) nature provides for this early nutrition. The prospective mother has in her body, if she is able to conceive, cells and tissues that are loaded with all the necessary nutrients. At first the mass of the developing embryo is very small and the *amount* of nutrition which needs to be supplied is also very minute. Later on, when the embryo weighs pounds instead of milligrams, the various nutrients must be supplied in substantial amounts.

All of the facts we have been citing point to the conclusion that in prenatal mammalian nutrition, as well as in nutrition at other stages, *there are many possible levels of excellence.* During the first few weeks of pregnancy, provided the prospective mother is reasonably well-nourished and doesn't contaminate her system with drugs, etc., the fetus usually encounters excellent nutrition, possibly the best it will encounter at any stage in its life. When the fetus becomes larger and requires a larger supply of all the nutrients, mild deficiencies and imbalances are liable to occur, and the nutrition is less excellent even though the baby, when born, may be judged to be superficially normal. As we have pointed out earlier, natural environments (including climates) are not, in general, perfectly adjusted to the needs of any organism.

Physicians are in the best position to judge how all these considerations impinge in a practical way on human prenatal nutrition. One dean of a medical school has written me, "Our human reproductive performance is terrible." How many other physicians would agree with this opinion I do not know. Physicians are more aware than any layman of the prevalence of developmental failures, deformities, etc., and how many of these may be attributed to mediocre nutrition.

My own feeling is that when it is frequently estimated that one baby in eight is mentally retarded, it is time to look at the problem of prenatal nutrition seriously and to ascertain whether poor or mediocre prenatal nutrition may not be largely responsible. There are so many potential ways in which the environment of growing fetuses can be deficient that it seems a major, but well worthwhile, project to find out how important, practically speaking, the quality of the prenatal environment is in human development.[5]

One of the most exciting findings made in recent years in the area of prenatal nutrition relates to prenatal brain development when female rats are forced by ligating one horn of the uterus to produce litters one-half the size they would otherwise be.[6] Under these conditions the brains of the newborn rats are larger and contain more cells, based on DNA determinations. The differences, about 10 percent, are highly significant statistically because of the importance of prenatal brain development. The quota of neurons, for example, is practically complete at birth in many mammals and, of course, these cells are not replaced when and if they are lost or worn out. It is possible that a baby rat or a human infant which does not have a fully adequate complement of brain cells at birth will be handicapped in this respect the rest of its life.

These findings strongly indicate that commonly experienced prenatal nutrition is indeed no different, in principle, from postnatal nutrition in that it is suboptimal and is capable of substantial improvement. The observations also suggest the possibility that in human beings multiple births may tend to lower the intellectual quality of the offspring. In the animal studies it was found that small litters, produced normally, were not associated with better developed brains, and it was concluded that only if the potential of the female exists will the brain size be increased by restricting the size of the litter. It would be interesting to know on the basis of statistical studies whether non-twins are superior intellectually to twins, and if super-intellects are found as often among twins as among non-twins.

Certainly these findings support the idea mentioned above that the birth of mentally retarded babies can probably be attributed largely though not exclusively to the poor or mediocre nutrition furnished by the mother to the growing fetus. That there should be concern about prenatal nutrition is supported by the material presented on page ii. This originated as a full page advertisement in many large newspapers and magazines under the sponsorship of the American Medical Association.

REFERENCES

1. Lefebvres-Biosselot, J.: Influence of slight pantothenic acid deficiency on the results of gestation. *Compt-Rend, Acad. Sci., Paris, 238*:2133, 1954.
2. Nelson, M.M., et al.: Multiple congenital abnormalties restulting from transitory pteroylglutamic acid deficiency during gestation in the rat. *J. Nutr., 56*:349, 1955.
3. Hale, F.: Pigs born without eyeballs. *J. Hered. 24*:105, 1935.
4. Williams, R.R. (Ed.): *Appraisal of Human Dietaries by Animal Experiment.* A Conference under the Auspices of the Williams Waterman Fund for the Combat of Dietary Diseases, Hotel Roosevelt, New York, 1947.
5. The relationship of nutrition to brain development and behavior. NAS-NRC Position Paper, Washington, D.C., 1973.
6. Van Marthens, E., and Zamenhof, S.: Desoxy-ribonucleic acid of neonatal rat cerebrum increased by operative restriction of litter size. *Exp. Neurol., 23*:214, 1969.

CHAPTER 7

BIOCHEMICAL INDIVIDUALITY

THE SUBJECT of this chapter is the title of a book written by the author and published by John Wiley & Sons in 1956.[1] I had the strong encouragement of my famous physician friend, Alan Gregg, M.D., Medical Director of the Rockefeller Foundation, who wrote the Foreword. This book has attracted sufficient attention so that it has been republished in two separate paperback editions and has been translated into Russian, Italian and Polish.

In my view the book is important not because it contains theories or speculations, but rather because it calls attention to *hard facts* regarding how *real people* are constituted. The wide range of highly significant variations which distinguish real people from hypothetical average people are anatomical, physiological, biochemical, neurological, endocrinological, psychological, etc. This book includes a compilation and presentation in one package of a vast amount of miscellaneous diverse material much of which has been known, in fragments, by physicians. The significance and meaning of the sum total of these facts (many of which were unbelievably striking) had, however, never received the serious attention of medical or biological scientists.

We can no longer delay a brief discussion of this material because it does impinge most importantly on the problems of nutrition. In the field of biochemistry where my particular interest centers, some of the variations among normal people are most astounding.

It is obvious that in two people of the same height and weight, the total energy metabolism (related to basal metabolic rate) is bound to be of the same order of magnitude and often approximately the same because such individuals carry the same weight when they move, have about the same body temperature, and have similar heat losses due to having about the same body surface area. The facts of biochemical individuality tell us, however, that in two young men with exactly the same basal metabolic rate, the *details of the burning process* may be enormously different. Specific chemical reactions involved in metabolism and induced by enzymes may take place ten or more times as rapidly in one of the individuals as in the other.

In summarizing the chapter on the normal differences of enzyme levels in blood and tissues, the following statement was made.

> The cumulative evidence that each individual human being has a distinctive pattern of enzyme efficiencies is hard to refute on any rational basis. Furthermore, inter-individual variation in enzyme efficiencies in normal individuals, insofar as they have been determined, are not of the order of 20 to 50 percent, but are more often at least three- or four-fold. Differences of ten- to fifty-fold have been observed in a substantial number of cases even when the number of normal individuals tested was small.[2]

That the digestive processes in different individuals are distinctive and strikingly different is indicated by the Mayo Clinic studies of the gastric juices of thousands of normal individuals. Both the pepsin content and the hydrochloric acid content were found to vary in healthy adults over at least a 100- to 200-fold range![3]

If we had comparably easy ways of finding out about the composition of intestinal and pancreatic juices, we would doubtless find substantial variations in these digestive juices too.[4,5] Indeed, in recent years it has been found that among normal healthy adults there is at least a ten- to 20-fold variation in the amounts of each of the three carbohydrate-splitting enzymes, lactase, sucrase and maltase, in the intestinal mucosa.[6] Such findings point to the probability that as more and more explorations are made, more and more striking evidence of biochemical individuality will be found. No one knows for sure, but the presumption is that the individual discrete specialized enzymes involved in protein digestion are unevenly distributed among the gastrointestinal tracts of the general population.

It would take far too much space to discuss in detail how biochemical individuality strikingly enters not only into the problems of digestion but also into absorption and the complicated interrelationships of intermediary metabolism. Suffice it to say at this time that the facts of biochemical individuality are to be found wherever we look for them and that the significance of these facts may be far reaching. My earlier book made a start toward elucidating these facts and their meaning.

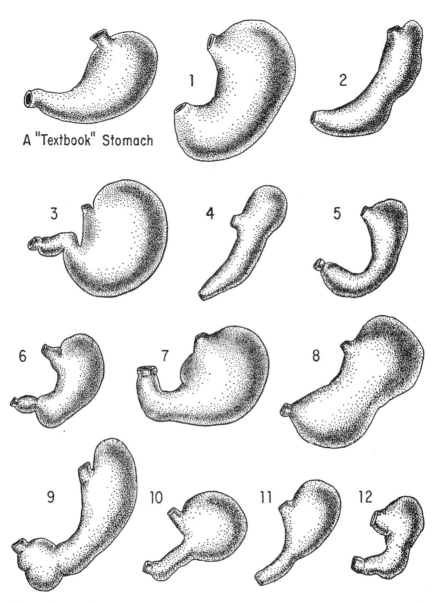

A "Textbook" Stomach

Gross Anatomical Variations in Human Stomachs (after Barry J. Anson's *Atlas of Human Anatomy*, W.B. Saunders Co., Philadelphia, 1951, p. 28, as published with permission in *You Are Extraordinary* by Roger J. Williams, Random House, New York, 1967. The figures 1-12 are drawings made from actual specimens. Gastric juices from different individuals vary far more in composition than stomachs do in size. See *Biochemical Individuality*, p. 60.)

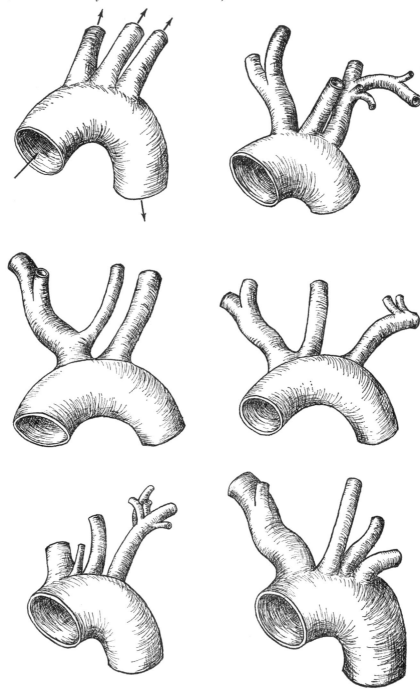

Physicians are in full agreement, I believe, that medicine is a blending of art and science, and that if it is considered a science, it is manifestly not a *pure* science but rather an *applied* science.

The ancient Hippocrates observed that "different sorts of people have different maladies" and Sir William Osler quoted with approval the old-time clinician, Parry of Bath, who held it to be "more important to know what sort of patient has a disease than to know what sort of disease a patient has." Clearly long-standing medical tradition completely supports a strong interest in individual patients and consequently in the question, "What *sorts* of people exist?"

If medicine were a pure science it would perhaps be interested in hypothetical average people. Being an applied science, its interest must be in real people who are of many sorts and suffer from many sorts of diseases. Only by paying attention to their biochemical individuality can one focus on the internal biochemistry of real people, all of whom are individuals.

The scientific basis of medical practice has changed markedly since the days of Sir William Osler or even Alan Gregg. Had these men been interested in what sorts of patients exist, there was comparatively little they could have done about it. Today, however, with the rapidly increasing development of automated equipment to analyze many entities not even recognized a decade or so ago, there is a great deal that can be done. New mathematical tools and computer techniques make possible the handling and storage of data with remarkable facility. Pertinent data with respect to distinctive individuals can be stored and used, and this practice will doubtless increase most significantly so that the leanings of individuals toward specific diseases can be studied (propetology).[7]

All of this impinges in a most pointed way on the problems of nu-

◀

Gross Variations in the Branching at the Aortic Arch (after Barry J. Anson's *Atlas of Human Anatomy*, W.B. Saunders Co., Philadelphia, 1951, p. 197 as published with permission in *You Are Extraordinary* by Roger J. Williams, Random House, New York, 1967. The upper left picture represents about 65% of observed cases. It is apparent from examination of Anson's extensive work that the variation in branching and artery sizes seen here, exemplifies similar differences in every organ and structure of the body.)

trition and the possibility of using nutritional means to support, maintain and restore health.

Just as each species of organism requires for its well-being a particular type of environment which is able to furnish to that species all of its essential needs, so also each individual person requires for his or her well-being an environment which will furnish all of his or her needs.

Each individual has a distinctive food environment problem of his or her own, because while the list of nutrients needed by all of us human beings may be the same, the respective amounts needed are necessarily not the same for all individuals. This is inevitable if differences in the enzyme efficiencies in different individuals exist.

These valid questions naturally arise: *"How distinctive* is the food-environment problem of each of us?" "Is this distinctiveness merely of academic interest, or does it have practical importance in daily life and health?" Rather than attempt to answer such questions in a dogmatic fashion, we will cite pertinent facts which will help each physician-reader to answer them to his own satisfaction.

Reasonably satisfactory definitive information is available regarding the variation in adult human needs for about nine of the nearly forty nutrients which we human beings need to obtain from our nutritional environment. These data are tabulated below.

Nutrient	Ranges of Needs by Adults	No. Subjects
Tryptophan[8, 9]	82 mg- 250 mg (3 fold)	50
Valine[8, 10]	375 mg- 800 mg (2.1 fold)	48
Phenylalanine[8, 11]	420 mg-1100 mg (2.6 fold)	38
Leucine[8, 12]	170 mg-1100 mg (6.4 fold)	31
Lysine[8, 13, 14]	400 mg-2800 mg (7 fold)	55
Isoleucine[8, 15]	250 mg- 700 mg (2.8 fold)	24
Methionine[8, 14]	800 mg-3000 mg (3.7 fold)	29
Threonine[8, 16]	103 mg- 500 mg (4.8 fold)	50
Calcium[17]	222 mg-1018 mg (4.6 fold)	19

It should be noted that the data for calcium apply to nineteen healthy young men and the amino acid data apply to a limited number of men and women. Presumably, if the data were collected from larger population samples the range of variation would be larger.

These data were all obtained from balance studies on individuals. Individuals cannot maintain a calcium balance unless adequate calcium is in the diet, and nitrogen equilibrium cannot be maintained in an individual unless each of the essential amino acids is furnished in adequate amounts. As as result, balance studies can be carried out, and they yield consistent numerical results. That these results are not the same for different individuals is, of course, a reflection of their biochemical individuality.

The data with respect to the vitamin A needs of human beings are very far from satisfactory though there are many interesting observations which throw some light on the problem. This problem has a long history, one phase of which began over forty years ago when Mead-Johnson and Company offered a large award to any investigator (or investigators) who "determines the vitamin A requirements of human beings."[18] This was one of three questions about vitamin A which were stated as the basis for the award. Thirteen years later, after four of the seven original judges were deceased, the judges advised the donors to withdraw the award on the basis that "it is their considered opinion that no report or reports have been published which adequately answer any of the three stated requirements of the Award—No adequate answers to the problems as formulated will result from current research."[19]

How can this shameful exhibition of investigative impotency be explained? There are a number of factors, but in my opinion the overriding reason is the fact that biochemical individuality is exhibited here to an astounding if not alarming degree. The needs of individuals vary so enormously that no single unifying assessment can possibly be made. How or why this extremely wide variation can exist is wholly unknown.

In the Sheffield Experiment in England about twenty years ago, one adult individual was kept on a diet virtually free of vitamin A for twenty-two months without exhibiting signs of deficiency.[20] In the light of the facts of biochemical individuality this observation unfortunately gives no clue as to how his neighbors (or young people) would have responded if they had received the same treatment. It is possible that this particular individual had comparatively a very large amount of vitamin A stored in his liver at the start of the experiment.

In the author's laboratory, a fresh attempt was made in 1966 by employing over 200 rats of four strains to determine the vitamin A needs of laboratory rats.[22] As a result of this study it was concluded

Because of the very large inter-individual differences it is not possible, using one or several criteria, to establish what the vitamin A needs of a rat strain are. Much less would it be possible to assess the needs of experi-

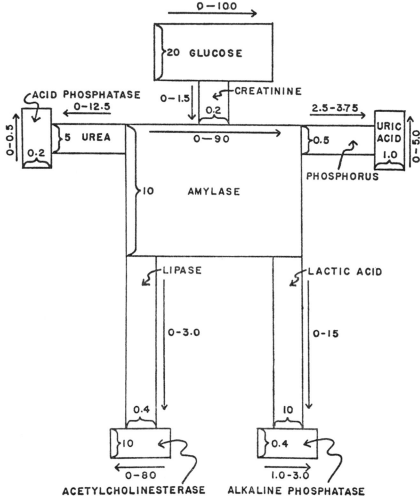

"Normal" Blood. This diagramatic representation depicts partially the characteristics of "normal" blood. The average amount and "normal" variation of each of eleven blood constituents is represented by a rectangle. The longer dimension, indicated by an arrow, represents the average level, and the shorter dimension, indicated by a brace, represents the "normal" extent of variation. The scales are so adjusted as to present a reasonably proportioned diagramatic picture of a man. From "Individual Patterns in Normal Humans: Organic Blood Constituents" by W. Duane Brown, Doctoral Dissertation, The University of Texas, 1955.

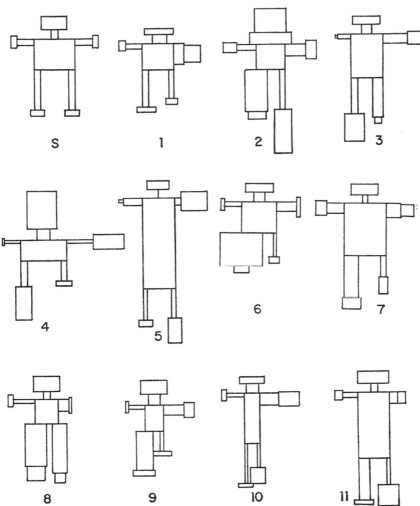

"Normal" Blood Variations. These diagramatic representations depict certain compositional levels in the fasting bloods of 11 healthy young men, in comparison with the "normal" or standard blood depicted on the opposite page. The levels and variations depicted for these 11 individuals were determined experimentally from 5 to 6 fasting blood samples from each, collected at about weekly intervals. These diagrams are reduced versions; the originals were drawn on exactly the same scale as that picturing "normal" blood. These representations appeared with permission in *You Are Extraordinary* by Roger J. Williams (Random House, New York, 1967) p. 22. They originated in "Individual Patterns in Normal Humans: Organic Blood Constituents" by W. Duane Brown, Doctoral Dissertation, The University of Texas, 1955.

mental rats generally . . . On the basis of satisfactory weight gains, some young rats appear to have sufficient vitamin A at the level of 0.4 units per gram of diet; on the other hand, some on the same diet failed to grow comparably at the 10 unit per gram level or even at the 50 unit per gram level.

It is obvious from the extensive experiments that have been carried out with vitamin A over several decades that the variation in rat needs is not a mere 25 percent, 50 percent or 100 percent but much larger, perhaps forty-fold or more.[23]

The problem of vitamin A requirements is complicated by the toxic effects at very high levels (at least when some preparations are used), and also by the fact that the functions of vitamin A, aside from those involved in vision, are totally unknown. Vitamin A acid, which cannot be used to produce visual pigments, can function in other parts of the body where it (or vitamin A itself) is absolutely essential in some unknown way to the health of epithelial tissues and, most significantly, to the entire reproductive process.[24]

It is most interesting to note on the basis of Bessey's competent estimations that *for groups of rats* normal visual thresholds are maintained when they receive 25 mcg per kg body weight per day, but that for maximum production of young 480 mcg per kg per day is needed. This nearly twenty-fold variation in the needs for different functions emphasizes the importance of cellular nutrition and *internal nutrition* as discussed in Chapter 5.[25]

We have already alluded to the evidence indicating that vitamin C needs vary greatly from one individual to another and that certainly wide variation exists in the vitamin C needs of the individuals in a guinea pig population. We will not discuss in detail the interindividual variations of human needs for other nutrients. There are indications, at least, that such variation is high in the cases of vitamin B_6, vitamin B_{12}, and vitamin D, but these do not stand alone. Interindividual variation of significant magnitude probably exists with respect to the needs for each essential nutrient.

A clear-cut exhibition of biochemical and nutritional individuality occurred when in our laboratory we fed sixty-four weanling rats of four strains an exclusive diet of white bread.[22]

The individual life spans on this diet ranged from six days up to 144 days, and the weight gains from two grams up to 212 grams. That these widely ranging results were not obtained because a few freak-ish individual rats were included in our experiment is shown by the examples of life spans and weight gains exhibited by a sampling of the individual rats, as listed below.

Life Spans on Bread Diet (in days): 6, 10, 11, 16, 20, 33, 34, 53 . . . . . . 69, 75, 87, 87, 110, 113, 122, 144.

Total Weight Gains on Bread Diet (in grams): 2, 10, 10, 23, 33, 40, 42, 64 . . . . . . 77, 85, 97, 98, 140, 155, 186, 212.

The vast subject of inborn individuality has a sound and unmis-takable biological basis. The entire evolutionary process could not have taken place if it did not exist, and it seems likely that the speed with which evolution can take place may be determined by the de-gree to which individuality exists. We have found in our laboratory that even monozygous quadruplet armadillos show, in some in-stances, wide inter-individual variation.[26] This goes to show that in-heritance of individual traits involves factors other than the com-monly considered nuclear genes. Even when these genes are pre-sumably identical, the animals show variation. It is interesting that the widest variation observed was in the area of biochemistry: hor-mone levels in glands and amino acid levels in the brains.

A sober view of the whole nutritional problem emphasizes the possibility if not the certainty that each individual, for maximum well-being, must have a total environment, including the assortment of nutrients derived from food, that is uniquely suitable for himself or herself. From what we have revealed about individuality, these distinctive needs are not based merely on hair-splitting differences.

No one can blame a busy practicing physician who is continually helping people in a practical way if he or she takes expedient short-cuts and tends to neglect individuality and individual differences when possible. Assuming the role of a prophet, the author is of the opinion, however, that more and more, especially in treating diseases of obscure etiology, physicians will have to consider thoroughly in-dividual metabolic profiles. The time will come, I think, when phy-sicians will, when they are freshly confronted with a patient, think *first* "What can be wrong with this individual's environment, in-cluding his nutritional environment, that could contribute to his or her condition?" The more that is known about biochemical individ-uality, the more likely this is to occur.

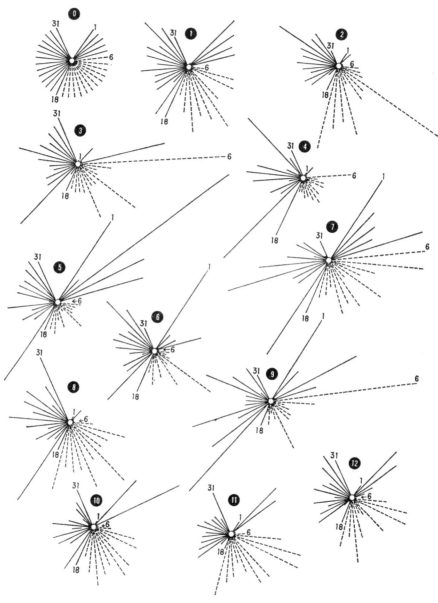

Individual Biochemical Patterns. Each radial line in these diagrams represents a separate type of measurement: (1-5) Taste sensitivities; creatinine, sucrose, KCl, NaCl, HCl (6-17) Salivary constituents; uric acid, glucose, leucine, valine, citrulline, alanine, lysine, taurine, glycine, serine, glutamic acid, aspartic acid (18-31) Urinary constituents; citrate, base R_F .28, acid

Continuing my role as a prophet, I will predict that physicians will in the future talk less and think less in terms of "the normal person" or "the average individual." There is such a multitude of ways in which a person can be normal or average, and an equal number of ways in which he or she can disconform or be a deviant that the terms "normal person" or "average person" are about as meaningless as would be the expressions "normal book," "average book," "normal painting," or "average tapestry."

The question of the meaning of the expression "normal value" has recently been discussed, and it is doubtful whether the so-called "normal values" commonly accepted, can generally stand the light of critical examination.[27] Certainly a value should not necessarily be designated as "normal" because it is exhibited by an individual who appears superficially to be well.

Inborn individuality is widely significant. There are different *sorts* of people, just as there are different sorts of books and paintings, and it is quite unscientific to fail to recognize this fact.

REFERENCES

1. Williams, R.J.: *Biochemical Individuality*. Austin, U of Tex Pr, 1973.
2. Williams, R.J.: *Biochemical Individuality*. Austin, U of Tex Pr, 1973, p. 77.
3. Osterberg, A.E., et al.: Pepsin in human gastric juice III: Physiologic aspects. *Am. J. Dig. Dis. 3*:35, 1936.
4. Rissel, E., and Wewalke, F.: Investigations of free amino acids in duodenal juice by paper chromatography I. *Klin. Wochenschr., 30*: 1065, 1952.
5. Rissel, E. and Wewalke, F.: Investigation of free amino acids in duodenal juice by paper chromatography II. *Klin. Wochenschr, 30*:1069, 1952.
6. Newcomer, A.D., and McGill, D.B.: Disaccharidase activity in small intestine: Prevalence of lactase deficiency in 100 healthy subjects. *Gastroenterology, 53*:881, 1967.
7. Williams, R.J., and Siegel, F.L.: Propetology, a new branch of medical science. *Am. J. Med., 31*:325, 1961.
8. Rose, W.C.: Amino acid requirements. *Nutr. Abstr. Rev.* 27:631, 1957.

R_F .32, gonadotropin, pH, pigment/creatinine, chloride/creatinine, hippuric acid/creatinine, creatinine, taurine, glycine, serine, citrulline, alanine. Each line represents the average of a series of determinations on each individual. Figures 1-12 represent different healthy individuals, including one pair of monozygous twins (11, 12). Figure 0 is the patternless hypothetical "average" or "normal." University of Texas Publication No. 5109 (1951) pp. 10-12.

9. Leverton, R.M., et al.: The quantitative amino acid requirements of young women III tryptophane. *J. Nutr., 58*:219, 1956.

10. Leverton, R.M., et al.: The quantitative amino acid requirements of young women II valine. *J. Nutr. 58*:83, 1956.

11. Leverton, R.M., et al.: The quantitative amino acid requirements of young women IV phenylalanine, with and without tyrosine. *J. Nutr. 58*:341, 1956.

12. Leverton, R.M., et al: The quantitative amino acid requirements of young women V leucine. *J. Nutr., 58*:355, 1956.

13. Jones, E.M., et al.: Nitrogen balance of women maintained on various levels of lysine. *J. Nutr. 60*:549, 1957.

14. Tuttle, S.G., et al.: Further observations on the amino acid requirements of older men II methionine and lysine. *Am. J. Clin. Nutr., 16*:229, 1965.

15. Swendseid, M.E.. et al.: Amino acid requirements of young women based on nitrogen balance data I the sulfur-containing amino acids. *J. Nutr., 58*:495, 1956.

16. Leverton, R.M., et al.: The quantitative amino acid requirements of young women I threonine. *J. Nutr., 58*:59, 1956.

17. Steggerda, F.R., and Mitchell, H.H.: Variability of calcium metabolism and calcium requirements of adult human subjects. *J. Nutr., 31*:407, 1946.

18. Williams, R.J.: *Biochemical Individuality*. Austin, U of Tex Pr, 1973, p. 143.

19. Advertisement in J.A.M.A., October 2, 1945.

20. Moore, T.: *Vitamin A*. Amsterdam, Elsevier, 1957, p. 368.

21. Hume, E.M., and Krebs, H.A.: *Med. Res. Counc. Spec. Rep. Ser.* (Lond.), No. 264, 1949.

22. Williams, R.J., and Pelton, R.B.: Individuality in nutrition: Effects of vitamin A deficient and other deficient diets on experimental animals. *Proc. Natl. Acad. Sci. USA, 55*:126, 1966.

23. Williams, R.J.: *Biochemical Individuality*. Austin, U of Tex Pr, 1973.

24. Moore, T.: Reproductive abnormalties. New York, Acad Pr, 1967.

25. Bessey, Otto: Personal communication. Graph reproduced in *Biochemical Individuality*, p. 146.

26. Storrs, E.E., and Williams, R.J.: A study of monozygous quadruplet armadillos in relation to mammalian inheritance. *Proc. Natl. Acad. Sci. USA, 60*:910, 1968.

27. Symposium: A New Look at Normal Values. Silver Anniversary Meeting of the American Association of Clinical Chemists in New York City, July 20, 1973.

CHAPTER 8

THE RANGE OF POTENTIAL BENEFITS TO BE DERIVED FROM THE IMPROVEMENT OF NUTRITIONAL ENVIRONMENTS: A NEW CONCEPT IN PATHOLOGY: GENERALIZED CYTOPATHY

FROM MY PHYSICIAN FRIENDS I want to beg indulgence if in this chapter I occasionally enter into speculations. Speculations should not be resisted or condemned except when they appear senseless or are presented in the guise of authentic information. We will continue to differentiate between what is fact and what is speculative.

We will find it profitable, I believe, to look into the question, "What kinds of benefits can *possibly* accrue from the perfect adjustment of the internal environment of cells?" To consider this, we must call upon all we know about biology and how cells operate and interact. We must recognize, of course, that this goal of a perfectly adjusted environment may be difficult to attain. It should certainly not be taken for granted that such an adjustment is simple or easy. The kind of adjustments and effects we may bring into our discussion should pave the way for advances that probably lie over the horizon of present-day practice.

Let us first look critically at some of the structures of the body where harmful effects are known to be brought about by poor cellular nutrition. There are already a great many evidences, including those derived from animal study, that the skin is vulnerable to nutritional lacks. In human pellagra, for example, there is the characteristic dermatitis which commonly accompanies this disease and vanishes when the individual with pellagra is cured. In animals when *biotin* deficiency is induced, a pathological skin condition occurs, and when the biotin deficiency is corrected the skin lesions disappear. Because of these observations, biotin was at one time called vitamin *H*, the H standing for the German word *Haut* or skin.

Deficiency of vitamin B_6 in rats induces a skin condition which has sometimes been called "rat pellagra" which again disappears when the missing vitamin is supplied in adequate amounts.

The first evidence that the cell nutrient on which I had worked for many years, pantothenic acid, is really a vitamin came with the demonstration that pantothenic acid will alleviate and cure what was called "chick dermatitis." Chickens suffering from this condition have most unhealthy skin and feathers, a condition which is clearly manifest.

The skin, partly because the circulation does not supply it with copious nutrition, is notoriously sensitive to nutritional lacks. In the oral cavity—the tongue, lips and the gums—we find a favorite region where nutritionists look to detect evidence of malnutrition.

When in our laboratories many years ago we explored further the condition chick dermatitis we found that the "skin deep" approach was far from adequate because this disease involved far more than the skin. Utilizing microbiological methods we were able to study biochemical lesions in other tissues, and it turned out that chick dermatitis, in addition to being a skin disease, was also a blood disease, a muscle disease, a liver disease, a kidney disease, and a disease of the spinal cord and of the brain. Not only were these tissues biochemically deficient with respect to their enzyme systems, but they exhibited this deficiency by being severely stunted.

The blood carried only one-fourth the usual amount of this nutrient; as a result, the livers and kidneys were less than half their usual size, the leg muscle mass was one-fourth its usual size, and the size of the brain and the spinal cord were decreased by 16 percent and 29 percent, respectively.

The biochemical lesions were such that the amount of pantothenic acid that could be extracted from a *unit weight* of tissue (stunted though the tissues were) was decreased 38 percent, 31 percent, 58 percent, 53 percent and 69 percent respectively in the five tissues: liver, kidney, muscle, brain and spinal cord.

It is notable that every tissue that was tested suffered severely, and to a somewhat characteristic degree; also that every tissue retained a substantial supply of this vital building block, otherwise it would not have been able to maintain its life as a tissue.[1]

It is obvious also that tissues can suffer to greatly varying degrees. Pantothenic acid deficiency is not an "all or none" matter, and mild deficiency would be expected to result in impairment of function but not complete incapacitation. Even in these chickens which were severely deficient, the livers, kidneys, muscles, brain and spinal cord were still functioning in a limited way.

Since every tissue examined was more or less severely diseased biochemically, it seems a reasonable extrapolation to conclude that every other tissue in the entire animal would have exhibited some deficiency if it had been examined. (Pantothenic acid is known to be an essential part of the machinery of every kind of cell.) If this conclusion is valid, chick dermatitis, in addition to being a disease of the blood, liver, kidney, muscle, brain and spinal cord, is also a disease of the heart, lung, gizzard, intestines, spleen, endocrine glands, the organs of the special senses, the reproductive system, and in fact of every cell and tissue in the body of the chicken. Correspondingly, pantothenic acid deficiency in mammals would also cause biochemical lesions in every cell and tissue. This interpretation and deduction is borne out by the following list of extremely diverse pathological conditions which have been observed in different species as a result of pantothenic acid deficiency: dermatitis,[1,2] keratitis,[3] ulceration throughout the gastrointestinal tract,[4,5] intussusceptions,[5,6] anemia[7,8,9] achromotrichia,[10] depigmentation of tooth enamel,[11,12] sterility,[13,14] congenital malformations,[15,16] bowel atony,[17,18] failure to produce antibodies,[19,20,21,22] hemorrhagic adrenal medulla and cortex,[23,24] spinal cord lesions,[26] dehydration,[24] fatty liver,[27] thymus involution,[11] kidney damage,[24,27] heart damage,[1,24,25] sudden death without warning,[27] bone marrow hypoplasia,[9] leucocyte deficiency,[7,9] spinal curvature,[28] myelin degeneration,[26] uncoordinated gait,[29,30] decreased longevity,[31] allergies,[32] headache,[22] loss of memory,[33] decreased resistance to stress.[9,34]

A careful consideration of these facts and the seemingly valid extrapolations we have made leads us to recognize pantothenic acid deficiency as leading to not only a systemic disease but to a generalized cytopathy, capable of damaging and incapacitating any and every structure in the entire body. This generalized cytopathy is an entirely different kind of disease than any which I have seen described in treatises on pathology.

Whether mild cases of generalized cytopathy can be detected by anatomical examination remains to be ascertained. It seems probable that electron microscope studies, at least, might reveal mild biochemical lesions. Whether such lesions are visible anatomically or not or can be made so, they are very real and can lead ultimately to the death of the cells and the entire organism.

On the basis of the facts discussed in the area of biochemical individuality, it is to be expected that *in different individuals* the same limited pantothenic acid intake might produce very different outward symptoms. Some individuals might be affected little because they have a relatively low requirement; others may be affected greatly because they have high requirements. Furthermore, the dominant lesions produced in two individuals would not be expected to be the same. Because individuals' circulatory systems, internal organ structures, and patterns of metabolism are highly distinctive, there is a wide range of possible damage from pantothenic acid deficiency, and no two individuals would be expected to suffer the same damage.

No one unacquainted with these considerations can be in a position to diagnose or pinpoint pantothenic acid deficiency or to tell whether or not it exists. It has been a source of annoyance to me that it has often been concluded that since pantothenic means "from everywhere" that shortages of this nutrient can never exist. Whether or not shortages exist depends on *supply* and *demand*. The supply is truly very widely distributed, but if the demand is higher than the available supply, shortages do exist.

That human beings are characteristically vulnerable to a shortage of pantothenic acid due to a relatively high requirement is indicated by certain compositional facts. In human milk the ratio between the pantothenic acid content and the thiamin content is about twice as high as the corresponding ratio in cow's milk. The corresponding ratio with respect to human muscle is much higher than in the muscles of other animals, 10 times as high as in hog muscle.[35] Since thiamin deficiency in humans can occur, these figures suggest that pantothenic acid deficiency is certainly not ruled out. *All* of the pantothenic acid in human muscles (and comparatively, it is abundant) must have an exogenous origin.

Due to the general failure to recognize that pantothenic acid deficiency is the root of a generalized cytopathy capable of causing impairment of any body structure, the possible existence of mild pantothenic acid deficiency in man has never received adequate attention. It has been estimated that if adults eat good wholesome food they get about 10 milligrams per day.[36] Whether some need as little as 5 mg per day and others need 25 mg or more a day for best performance is not known. It is clear from experimental work with animals that they may have deficiencies which range all the way from very mild (certainly not outwardly noticeable) up to severe, and that mild deficiencies can exist even when the animals appear to be relatively healthy.

That mature hens on ordinary diets, for example, may often be experiencing mild pantothenate deficiency is shown by the fact that the hatchability of their eggs may be very significantly increased by supplementing their diet with extra pantothenate.[37]

That mature rats may suffer from mild pantothenate deficiency and yet appear outwardly healthy is shown by the fact that on ordinary diets they often have poor reproductive records and certainly, as an earlier discussion has shown, pantothenate deficiency is one of the important factors that may be involved.

That adult mice on a chow diet continuously may live with a pantothenic acid deficiency is shown by an experiment we performed several years ago when we carried out a study of the effect of extra dietary pantothenic acid on the longevity of mice. Two groups of mice were fed the same commercial chow; one group was supplied with water, the other group received water to which had been added a small amount of calcium pantothenate such that the mice would each receive about 300 micrograms per day.

The results of the experiment were that the animals receiving the extra pantothenic acid lived on the average about 19 percent longer. This was highly significant statistically and showed that the mice receiving the chow diet were somewhat impaired by a mild pantothenic acid deficiency. This is more significant because the chow diet was considered a fully adequate one *supposedly well-supplied* with pantothenic acid.

I would be willing to wager that if a similar experiment were done with human beings the results would be comparable. My willingness to gamble on this is enhanced by the evidence that human beings are probably unusually susceptible to pantothenic acid deficiency. One way to test this hypothesis would be to determine the effects, if any, of extra pantothenic acid on the reproductive performance of pregnant women. A controlled experiment of this sort would not be very involved or expensive.

The existence of such a pathology as generalized cytopathy capable of affecting any tissue, is broadly important because further reflection leads to the conclusion that there are potentially many examples of such disease.

Pellagra, sometimes linked to the four D's—dermatitis, diarrhea, dementia and death—is probably such a disease. Niacinamide is an essential part of the energy-metabolism machinery of every cell in one's body. When one is deficient in niacinamide the functioning of every cell must be impaired to a greater or lesser degree. Whether the overt symptoms show up on the skin or in a pathological intestinal tract or in the brain is somewhat incidental to the probability that pellagra exemplifies a generalized cytopathy, incapacitating each and every tissue.

To the best of our present knowledge all the well-recognized B vitamins such as thiamin, riboflavin, niacinamide, pantothenic acid, folic acid, biotin, vitamin B_6 and vitamin B_{12} are essential cogs in the machinery of all mammalian cells. A deficiency of any one of these probably induces a characteristic generalized cytopathy. That this is so is indicated by the fact that mental symptoms, for example, are reportedly associated with deficiencies of each and every one of these vitamins. It seems probable that when one suffers from beriberi, pellagra, macrocytic anemia or pernicious anemia, every cell and tissue in the body is impaired.

The nutritionally essential amino acids are also to the best of our knowledge necessary for the functioning of all kinds of cells, and their deficiency also should lead to generalized cytopathy capable of impairing any and every tissue.

The minerals, including the trace minerals, are likewise needed by all cells, and their deficiency should also produce characteristic generalized cytopathies. Calcium deficiency, to take one familiar example, would of course lead to bone depletion, but there are many enzyme systems which depend on calcium, and every cell in the body would be ultimately affected by a calcium lack.

For the other vitamins A, C, E, D, K, the situation is not clear, simply because the functions of these nutrients are imperfectly known. It is not even known, for example, that each of these vitamins is needed by every cell. Vitamin A (or vitamin A acid) is probably very widely needed, but perhaps not by every cell. Vitamin C is certainly widely needed for structural reasons (collagen building) but again we have no knowledge that every cell needs it. Similar doubts exist with respect to the other vitamins not in the B group. This does not in any way detract from their importance, but it does make it clear that the pathology incident to their deficiency may be distinctly different from that of a generalized cytopathy.

If and when we admit the existence of a series of generalized cytopathies, we have answered the question of the potential range of nutritional benefits. All disorders which have a cellular origin are included among those which can presumably be ameliorated by improving cellular nutrition. This statement covers a lot of territory because the cell is the unit of life, and every functioning part of our bodies is built up of cells.

There is one area of our cellular anatomy which needs badly to be considered in this connection, the cells of the nervous system. Psychiatrists, in whose domain lie the mental diseases, often speak a foreign tongue so far as other physicians are concerned. The non-biologically oriented psychiatric specialists remain habitually oblivious to the vital cellular physiology and biochemistry involved in mental activity. This probably seems to them a routine process which can be neglected because it takes place automatically, regardless of circumstances. There are growing numbers of biologically oriented psychiatrists, however, who realize that there must be physiologically and biochemically something wrong in the brains of mentally ill people. For these psychiatrists two new organizations have been formed in recent years: the Academy of Orthomolecular Psychiatry, and the Society of Biologic Psychiatry. For physicians with more general interest there are two new organizations, The International Academy of Preventive Medicine and the International

Academy of Metabology, Inc. An older organization with similar interests is the International College of Applied Nutrition.

It has been estimated on the basis of cell counts involving the brains of those who have died at different ages that on the average an adult's brain cells die off at a rate of 1,000 to 2,000 cells per hour. Biologically oriented psychiatrists may be inclined to ask *why* these cellular deaths occur. Even if it is granted that there is an inevitable aging process, the questions remain: "Do not brain cells die because their environments become unsuitable?" and "Cannot improving the nutritional environment of these brain cells prolong their life and effectiveness?" It is certainly an open question whether all mental disease may not have as its basis a derangement of cellular metabolism. Is it not to be expected that every type of generalized cytopathy can be capable of producing mental disease?

The concept of generalized cytopathy capable of deranging any cell system in the body falls in line with biologically oriented psychiatry. It also makes it possible to view many unusual health-related experiences that individual people may have with far more understanding.

Physicians are justifiably extremely unwilling to accept at face value any wild-eyed testimonial from uninformed persons. They have also learned even to mistrust other physicians when they become enthusiastic about some treatment which doesn't seem to make sense. There has developed among medically trained personnel a most urgent desire to see the results of a *controlled* experiment before seriously considering the possible advantages of any unfamiliar treatment.

In spite of my recognition of this skepticism and my complete sympathy with it, I wish to present and comment on, for the consideration of my physician-readers, a series of individual experiences which need to be considered *in the light of the earlier discussions in this chapter.* Out of this context these incidents may be relatively meaningless, inconsequential or even misleading.

A science professor in one of our most highly regarded institutions came to me with a story of his experience with what was diagnosed as *psoriasis.* For this condition he tried taking rather heavy doses (about 25,000 units daily) of vitamin A. After some months the rash disappeared and continued to be absent. He was subsequently called to a foreign country on a scientific mission and found it difficult to obtain supplies of vitamin A. Months later the "psoriasis" condition reappeared. He came back to this country shortly and experimented with himself using intermittent trials. He became convinced that extra vitamin A intake prevented the condition and that failure to ingest the extra vitamin A caused the condition to recur.

These observations, if taken at their face value, of course, do not prove that psoriasis is cured by vitamin A, but they do indicate that the condition with which this scientist was afflicted, whatever it was, was banished by vitamin A administration. In the light of our earlier discussions, including those related to *biochemical individuality*, the concept of generalized cytopathy and our lack of knowledge about how vitamin A functions, this observation becomes credible. Without these concepts, it probably is not.

On another occasion a woman physician came to my office to discuss with me what seemed at the time a rather outlandish observation she had made with respect to her own eyesight. She found, by trial and error, that the impairment of her vision and her inability to use her eyes for continuous reading was completely remedied when she administered to herself daily a generous dose of thiamin or vitamin B_1.

This observation, again if taken at face value, does not by any means prove that eyesight troubles should be treated with thiamin, but it does, *in the light of our discussion*, suggest that the functioning of the eyesight mechanism may sometimes be impaired by a thiamin lack. It also suggests that some individuals (specifically this physician) have a relatively high requirement for this particular vitamin. What particular cells may have suffered most from the deficiency I do not know. All retinal cells, for example, need thiamin for the metabolic processes which are associated with the regeneration of visual pigments.

A graduate student in psychology in one of my classes told me of quite a different eyesight experience which was related to nutrition. He was partially color-blind and had developed methods, by use of visual charts, of studying the degree to which this condition existed. Having heard of the close connection between vitamin A and visual pigments he began studying how extra vitamin A intake might affect his condition, if at all. While I cannot accept with complete confidence his findings, he became convinced that his color-blindness was partially abolished when he had a high intake of vitamin A.

If taken at its face value, his finding suggests that improvement of color vision (mild impairment is widespread) may sometimes be accomplished by giving the retinal cells involved a better nutritional environment.

Another observation involving eyesight symptoms as related to a nutritional factor was to me completely convincing. A young science professor was consistently and painfully bothered, particularly by bright fluorescent lights. His eyes were so sensitive to this type of glare that even though he wore a special green eyeshade at all times he considered, I am told, moving to a less advanced country where fluorescent lights were not yet in common use.

Knowing of another young man who had complained of being sensitive to glare and having this difficulty abolished by the administration of about 15 mg of riboflavin daily, I purposely encountered the young professor with the green eyeshade and suggested that he try taking some extra riboflavin. He started at the 5 mg a day level expecting to take more if the 5 mg failed to bring relief. Experience showed, however, that at the 5 milligram level his sensitivity disappeared completely. He discarded his eyeshade and for a period of years has had no further difficulty.

In this case again I have no adequate detailed explanation, but it seems clear that in his case sensitivity to glare was abolished. It seems probable that this young man had an inborn need for riboflavin that is higher than average.

On one occasion I had a visit from a retired army nurse who traveled from another city to tell me of her gratitude. She was overjoyed that she had received invaluable and unexpected benefit from ingesting daily extra pantothenate which she took for no particular reason other than that it was a newly available vitamin. Her completely unexpected findings were two-fold. First, the extra supply of this vitamin darkened her greying hair, and second, it improved *remarkably*, she thought, her failing memory.

She gave a rather convincing recital concerning what pantothenic acid had done for her memory. She had been retired prematurely from the army as a nurse *because* her memory was failing. She would forget what days or hours she was to be on duty. She would often show up when she was not expected and failed to appear when she was expected. Later, after her retirement and after she began taking pantothenic acid and modified her activities in no other way, her memory came back in what seemed to her a most striking way. This was illustrated when she was a passenger involved in an automobile accident, and was complimented after a court appearance for her clear-cut, detailed, and decisive testimony. She had remembered everything just as it happened.

This observation, if taken at its face value, does not prove that pantothenic acid will always improve failing memories, but the facts suggest that in this particular case it did accomplish this unexpected fact. Presumably, brain cells were furnished a better environment. Previous to her experience, unknown to her, some evidence had been found that pantothenic acid may benefit victims of Korsakoff's syndrome.

Another series of incidents involved a graduate student, now a professor. In traveling by car across the desert he had repeatedly become afflicted with allergy symptoms which disappeared when he left behind the desert area. On a hunch he tried dosing himself with 20 mg or more of pantothenic acid daily before one of his frequent trips. The result was an absence of allergy. He repeated the test both with and without pantothenic acid, always with consistent results. These and other observations were submitted to a pharmaceutical house for further exploration. Corroboration of his finding resulted, but the benefits were not consistent for all individuals, and the pharmaceutical house could find no way of exploiting the findings profitably, so the matter was dropped.

Scientifically, however, it seems entirely reasonable to conclude that in some individuals allergies can be prevented by administration of pantothenic acid alone. It does not require a very long leap of the imagination to conclude that probably in many other individuals similar benefits could be derived if the nutritional environment could be improved in other ways.

Still another observation involving pantothenic acid was made by a highly intelligent friend whom I have known almost from youth. This individual who had been a "life-long sufferer from constipation" told me that when extra pantothenic acid was taken regularly, this difficulty completely disappeared, but returned as soon as the use of the vitamin was discontinued. To this individual, pantothenic acid is a boon. This observation is perhaps related to the effective use in medicine of pantothenic acid in the treatment of *paralytic ileus.*

These three observations indicating that *in some cases* extra pantothenic acid may benefit failing memories and may abolish constipation and allergies, can be taken as evidence supporting the thesis that pantothenic acid deficiences do exist in the human family when ordinary food is consumed.

An interesting observation involving another kind of nutrient, an essential amino acid, was brought to my attention *confidentially* by a physician who was acquainted with the circumstances. I was not able to get full information and cannot properly identify the observation publicly because those involved wished to avoid publicity. A study was being made of the needs of a series of individuals for some of the essential amino acids. In order to do this, it was essential that certain individuals receive for a time diets relatively free from the amino acid under investigation. In one case where this was done, the individual showed alarming symptoms, particularly with respect to the teeth. Several teeth were involved, and when it was evident that serious trouble was ahead, it was necessary to terminate depriving this individual of the usual supply of this amino acid. The implications of this finding are obvious: "How often are teeth adversely affected by amino acid deficiencies?" No one knows.

In another study, at Purdue University, a group of volunteer students were being given diets low in lysine, one of the essential amino acids we have listed. One student had to withdraw from the experiment because his mental faculties began to fail; he could not concentrate and was in danger of failing his examinations. When the student was given adequate lysine, his nitrogen balance was restored, and his difficulties of concentration disappeared. This finding suggests a question to which there is no known answer: "How often are mental difficulties aggravated by mild amino acid deficiencies?" We have already noted that the lysine requirement of individuals varies at least seven-fold. (See p. 44, Ch. 7.)

The most bizarre observation in the area of nutrition that I have encountered was relayed to me by an officer of one of our largest New York foundations. A man given a comprehensive nutritional supplement was found to be completely relieved of a disorder not often discussed in medical circles, malodorous feet. The contrast, before and after, was so striking that it could not escape notice. The individual, after his dietary supplementation, was so free from this difficulty that he wore the same socks for four successive days, and at the end of this time they were reported to have no perceptible odor. This bit of information I have thought too outlandish to report until I received a completely independent unsolicited report of exactly the same thing from the family of a close friend who had never heard of such an observation before.

Of course, we know that body odors are the product of metabolism, and if nutritional adjustments can alter metabolism, there is no reason to suppose that body odors could not also be substantially altered.

Coming back to cases involving more acute pathology, let us consider a prominent lawyer in one of our larger cities who had a most gratifying experience in connection with the use of a comprehensive nutritional supplement. He had been rejected for life insurance a year before this experience because of high blood pressure. As a result of tests in a prominent clinic, he was advised to undergo a sympathectomy. He declined to do this and was then advised to use barbiturates to settle his nerves. He also began to drink heavily and became over a period of time intoxicated regularly, more than once a week. When he was admitted to a hospital he had no control over his drinking and was taking about fourteen 1½ grain Seconal® tablets per day.

The doctor who supervised his care had heard of our work involving the use of complex nutritional supplements for alcoholism and decided to give our recommendations a try. In a surprisingly short time the individual's condition improved markedly, and in a few weeks he left the hospital and returned to work. His blood pressure had dropped from 180/120 to 130/90, and he had no more craving for Seconal or for alcohol. I saw this man about a year later. He was in good health, had gained about twenty pounds (he was still slightly underweight according to the accepted tables), took the supplements regularly, took no Seconal, and drank socially only occasionally, and had no desire to drink more.

This case does not justify any conclusions regarding what can be done for all alcoholics or all barbiturate addicts or for all victims of high blood pressure. It does suggest, however, that all these conditions may at least occasionally be greatly ameliorated by the use of nutritional measures: wholesome food and intelligently compounded supplements to insure that a variety of nutrients will be received in abundant amounts.

While the nutritional approach to alcoholism was being initially explored, my colleague, Professor William Shive, discovered that glutamine (but not glutamic acid) would protect bacteria from alcohol poisoning.[38] Subsequently, we found that glutamine administration (but not that of glutamic acid or asparagine) would decrease statistically the voluntary consumption of alcohol by rats.[39] Following this, J. B. Trunnel, M.D., of Houston, Texas, told us of a case of an individual alcoholic who was treated with glutamine without the individual knowing that any treatment was being used. (Glutamine is tasteless.) The result was that in a short time the individual for no other apparent reason than an altered internal desire stopped drinking and has remained sober and became gainfully employed.

These examples of relief from alcoholism by nutritional means do not stand alone. Hundreds and even thousands have seemingly gained great benefit. Many side benefits such as freedom from headaches and from insomnia have also been reported. Glutamine is the only amino acid which readily passes the blood-brain barrier and is utilized by the brain cells; this lends credence to the idea that it may influence regulatory mechanisms in the brain. All the other nutrients also get to the brain cells (often less readily than glutamine), and the thousands who appear to have gained relief from the use of nutritional supplements point to the probability that alcoholism is primarily a disease of the brain cells. These observations need desperately to be confirmed or discarded on the basis of carefully controlled experiments.

Finally, I will report how in my own individual case mineral nutrients have brought benefits by improving my internal environment.

At the time this observation was made I had been taking an antibiotic to treat a bladder infection. This may have had something to do with the condition. At any rate, I developed night after night, without exception, severe cramps in my legs. Without going into great detail, I discovered that a generous slug of precipitated chalk from the laboratory abolished the cramps entirely beginning the first night after it was ingested. However, while not cramping, my legs felt very restless and uncomfortable. A blood analysis arranged by my doctor showed that my calcium level was relatively high. (This was not surprising since I had been taking calcium carbonate.) But my phosphate level was at a low level of "normality." Immediately I changed and began taking $CaHPO_4$ instead of calcium carbonate with the result that the uneasiness in my legs completely disappeared the first night after I took it, and my trouble has not returned. In my case, at least, the extra calcium and phosphate must have overcome shortages; they did abolish the severe cramps and put my legs at ease. What these nutrients will do for people generally I do not know. I do know of a few others who have had experiences similar to mine; in one case relief from severe incapacity to use the hands was obtained.

The contents of this chapter can be briefly summarized as follows: There has been developed a new concept in pathology, that of generalized cytopathies capable of impairing any and all functioning structures of the body. When and if such diseases can be prevented by nutritional manipulation, there are no limits to the kinds of benefits that can accrue. We have also cited individual cases where unusual or even bizarre disorders have seemingly been abolished by nutritionally improving the internal environments of the individuals concerned. The concept of generalized cytopathy helps in the understanding of these happenings, and because of the multitude of possible applications, further investigation in this vast area is very much in order.

REFERENCES

1. Snell, E.E., Pennington, D., and Williams, R.J.: Effect of diet on pantothenic acid content of chick tissues. *J. Biol. Chem.*, *133*:559, 1940.
2. Sheppard, A.J., and Johnson, B.C.: Pantothenic acid deficiency. *J. Nutr.*, *61*:195, 1957.
3. Bowles, L.L., Hall, W.K., Sydenstriker, V.P., and Hock, C.W.: Corneal changes in the rat with deficiencies of pantothenic acid and pyridoxine. *J. Nutr.*, *37*:9, 1949.
4. Berg, B.N., Zucker, T.F., and Zucker, L.M.: Duodenal ulcers produced on a diet deficient in pantothenic acid. *Proc. Soc. Exp. Biol. Med.*, *71*:374, 1949.

5. Hughes, E.H.: Pantothenic acid in the nutrition of the pig. *J. Agr. Res.,* *64*:185, 1942.

6. Hughes, E.H., and Ittner, N.R.: Minimum requirements of panothenic acid for the growing pig. *J. Anim. Sci.,* *1*:116, 1942.

7. Carter, C.W., MacFarlane, R.G., O'Brian, J.R.P., Robb-Smith, A.H.T., and Amos, B.: Anemia of nutritional origin in the rat. *Biochem. J. 39*:339, 1945.

8. McCurdy, P.: Is there an anemia responsive to pantothenic acid? *J. Am. Pediatr. Soc., 21*:88, 1973.

9. Dumm., M.E., Ovando, P., Roth, P., and Ralli, E.P.: Relation of pantothenic acid to white blood cell response of rats following stress. *Proc. Soc. Exp. Biol. Med., 71*:368, 1949.

10. Groody, T.C., and Groody, M.E.: Feather depigmentation and pantothenic acid deficiency in chicks. *Science, 95*:655, 1942.

11. Phillips, P.H., and Engel, R.W.: Chicks deficient in the chick antidermatitis factor or pantothenic acid. *J. Nutr., 18*:227, 1939.

12. Ziskin, D.E., Stein, G., Gross, P., and Runne, E.: Mouth conditions in rats under a low pantothenate diet with the addition of $ZnCO_3$ (Abstract) *J. Dent. Res., 23*:152, 1944.

13. Kratzer, F.H., Davis, P.N., Marshall, B.J., and Williams, D.E.: Pantothenic acid requirement of turkey hens. *Poult. Sci., 34*:68, 1955.

14. Barboriak, J.J., Krehl, W.A., Cowgill, F.R., and Whedon, A.D.: Effect of partial pantothenic acid deficiency on reproductive performance. *J. Nutr., 66*:457, 1958.

15. Lefebres-Biosselot, J.: Influence of slight pantothenic acid deficiency on the results of gestation. *Comptes Rend., 238*:2123, 1954.

16. Nelson, M.M., Wright, H.V., Baird, C.C., and Evans, H.M.: Teratogenic effects of pantothenic acid deficiency. *J. Nutr., 62*:395, 1957.

17. Schulte, F.J.: Die Wirkung des Beppenthau auf Tonus und Motilität des Darmes nach chirurgischen eingriffen. *Dtsch. Med. Wochenschr. 82*: 1188, 1957.

18. Nardi, G.L., and Zuidema, G.D.: The post-operative use of d-pantothenyl alcohol. *Surgery, 112*:526, 1961.

19. Ginunchi, G., et al.: The influence of some antibiotics on the growth and production of antibodies in rats fed a pantothenic acid deficient diet. *Exptl. Med. & Surg. 12*:430, 1954.

20. Ludovici, P.P., Axelrod, A.E., and Carter, B.B.: Circulating antibodies in vitamin deficiency states—pantothenic acid deficiency. *Proc. Soc. Exp. Biol. Med., 72*:81, 1949.

21. Zucker, T.F., and Zucker, L.M.: Pantothenic acid deficiency and loss of natural resistance to a bacterial infection in the rat. *Proc. Soc. Exp. Biol. Med., 85*:517, 1954.

22. Hodges, R.E., Bean, W.B., Ohlson, M.A., and Bleiler, R.E.: Immunogenic responses of men deficient in pantothenic acid III. Factors affecting human antibody response. *Am. J. Clin. Nutr., 11*:85, 1962.

23. Mills, R.C., et al.: Curative effects of pantothenic acid on adrenal necrosis. *Proc. Soc. Exp. Biol. Med., 45*:482, 1940.

24. Supplee, G.C., Bender, R.C., Kahlenberg, O.J., and Babcock, L.C.: Interrelated vitamin requirements—kidney damage, adrenal hemorrhage and cardiac failure correlated with inadequacy of pantothenic acid. *Endocrinology, 30*:355, 1942.

25. Smith, S.G.: Red staining of paws and whiskers in vitamin B complex deficient rats after dehydration. *Proc. Soc. Exp. Biol. Med., 49*:651, 1942.

26. Lippincott, S.W., and Morris, H.P.: Morphologic changes associated with pantothenic acid deficiency. *J. Natl. Cancer Inst., 2*:39, 1941.

27. Schaefer, A.E., McKibbin, J.M., and Elvejem, C.A.: Pantothenic acid deficiency studies in dogs. *J. Biol. Chem., 143*:321, 1942.

28. Sandza, J.G., and Cerecedo, L.R.: Requirement of the mouse for pantothenic acid and a new factor in the vitamin B complex. *J. Nutr., 21*:609, 1941.

29. Wintrobe, M.M., et al.: Prevention of sensory neuron degeneration—role of liver fractions. *J. Clin. Invest., 31*:710, 1942.

30. Hodges, R.E., Ohlson, M.A., and Bean, W.B.: Human pantothenic acid deficiency produced by omega-methyl pantothenic acid. *J. Clin. Invest., 37*:1642, 1958.

31. Pelton, R.B., and Williams, R.J.: Effect of pantothenic acid on longevity of mice. *Proc. Soc. Exp. Biol. Med., 49*:632, 1958.

32. Ershoff, B.H., and Slayter, R.B.: Effects of pantothenic acid deficiency on pituitary-adrenal function. *J. Nutr., 50*:299, 1953.

33. Gordon, B.S.: Pantothenic acid in human nutrition. In Evans, E.A. Jr. (Ed.): *Biological Action of the Vitamins.* Chicago, U of Chicago Pr, 1942, p. 186.

34. Ralli, R.P., and Dumm, M.E.: Nutritional fractions affecting survival of young adrenalectomized rats. *Vitam. Horm. 11*:135, 1953.

35. Biochemical Institute Studies II: Studies on the Vitamin Content of Tissue II, pp. 37-40, 41-56, 105-124, University of Texas Publication 4237, 1942.

36. Williams, R.J.: Approximate vitamin requirements of human beings. *J.A.M.A., 119*:1, 1942.

37. Taylor, A., Thacker, J., and Pennington, D.: The effect of increased pantothenic acid in the egg on the development of the embryo. *Science, 94*:542, 1941.

CHAPTER 9

THE ROLE OF NUTRITIONAL
SUPPLEMENTS

IF AND WHEN nutritional supplements are to be recommended, there should be an intelligent basis for doing so. It is not my purpose to try to decide for physicians whether or under what circumstances they will want to use nutritional supplements. Physicians are the qualified, trained experts on disease, and all I can do is to present some information and propound some questions which may help them decide wisely.

Recommendations for supplementing people's diets should be made with full recognition of the basic principles of nutrition, the purpose of nonfuel nutrition, the need for fundamental units which *acting as a team* make metabolism possible, the interdependence of all organisms, the cellular dependence on nutrition, the prevalence of suboptimal nutrition, and the universal individuality exhibited by all people. In addition to these nutritional principles, there are, of course, commonsense considerations such as availability and cost, ease of administration, palatability, etc.

Perhaps in no way have people in general exhibited the "nutritional illiteracy" (to borrow a phrase from H. J. Heinz, Jr.) more consistently than in the way they "take their vitamins."[1] One person, a former college president, was reported to me as having taken two tablets of vitamin B_6, thinking this was the same as vitamin B_{12}. If people start taking a widely publicized brand of vitamins, they are likely to continue (if at all) without reference to new developments or the contents of the preparation, so long as it is well advertised.

The use of supplements began when only a few vitamins had been discovered, and they were thought of as like magic wands.

Wand A, wand B, wand C and wand D gradually became availble for waving. With the advent of more knowledge about nutrients, their number, their functioning and their interrelations, there should have been a revolutionary change in attitude, but there has been a strong tendency to stick by the "old favorites."

In the 1940's the high priests and priestesses of nutrition thought the nutritional situation had settled down, and there were about six major concerns: vitamins A and D, thiamin, riboflavin, niacin and iron. Calcium, iodine and ascorbic acid were perhaps minor concerns. All these substances were available candidates for inclusion in nutritional supplements. The fact that four of these—thiamin, riboflavin, niacin and iron—were being added to bread and flour did not diminish their strong appeal; they were general favorites and were furnished in supplements, often as the principal ingredients.

Currently the entire list of known nutrients (minerals, trace minerals, amino acids and vitamins) needs to be brought into view when and if supplements are formulated, because every cog is an essential one, and there is no ruling out the importance of any nutrient.

The question of who, if anyone, should get nutritional supplements is vitally important. There are two questions which potentially may receive very different answers. The first is, "Should healthy people concentrate on eating good food and forget all about nutritional supplements?" And the second is, "Should those who are chronically afflicted with obscure disorders (major and minor) for which no adequate treatment is known also concentrate alone on eating good food and discard the idea of taking nutritional supplements?"

Physicians who may be inclined to say "Yes" to the first question might not be so willing to say "Yes" to the second. There are other questions, too, which may be answered differently by different physicians. "Are pregnancy and old age times when the use of nutritional supplements should receive favorable attention?"

To answer all these questions in their own minds, physicians will need to answer other questions such as, "How many people are fundamentally sound and healthy?" I have heard a definition of health which goes something like this, "Health is a completely disease-free condition, striven for but never attained." In the light of our discussion of the prevalence of suboptimal environments, does this definition make any sense? Does the government report that one out of three prospective inductees is unfit for military service throw light on the prevalence of significant disease in the general population?[2]

Other questions of a different nature also arise: How easy (or difficult) is it to get a balanced diet? Are balanced diets common or uncommon among those selected by the general population? Are there specific nutrients among the minerals, trace minerals, amino acids or vitamins which are difficult to get in adequate amounts from currently available foods? Are there "convenience foods" which need to be avoided if one is to get a well-balanced diet? Is there need for strict attention to the nutritional value of marketed foods on the part of food merchants? Is the staple food, "enriched" bread, as supplied to the general public suitable for dominant inclusion in a balanced diet?

One basic question needs to be considered if one assumes for the moment that nutritional supplements are to find some use: "What kinds of supplements should be available?" Probably we should use as a starting point a general supplement—one that could safely be taken by anyone—and one directed toward *helping insure* the individual who takes it against the deficiencies which need most to be guarded against.

The principle of insurance needs to be considered here. It can be argued that one does not buy fire insurance on his home because he knows it is going to burn down. Usually he is reasonably confident that it will not, but he can't be sure. In a parallel fashion a person who takes a nutritional supplement as insurance doesn't know that he is eating inadequately; he may think his diet is adequate, but he isn't *sure*, so he takes a nutritional supplement just in case.

A supplement designed to serve this purpose should, it seems, be broadly formulated to include everything that can conveniently be supplied without prohibitive cost. Following up our fire insurance analogy, one would not want to buy fire insurance which was *restricted*. Such restricted insurance, in order to remain in force, might stipulate, for example, that the fire has to be caused by a lighted cigarette. (If it is caused by a cigarette lighter, defective wiring, a leaky gas main or a multitude of other causes, the insurance would be void.) What we commonly insure against is fire starting in any way whatever. Similarly, a person buying nutritional insurance would like to be insured against any metabolic weakness whatever, not against one specific deficiency alone, like that of calcium, thiamin, iron, or some other single nutrient. He would wish to be insured, if possible, against all deficiencies.

It is not feasible to formulate a supplement of reasonable size and cost which will insure against *all* deficiencies. Several of the minerals and amino acids are required individually in amounts of from one-fourth gram up to several grams daily, and these amounts cannot readily be put into capsules or in solutions to be administered in limited amounts. Furthermore, supplements containing relatively large amounts of several minerals and amino acids would probably be harmful to some because they would probably contribute to a poor balance. General supplements, for reasons of practicality, must be limited largely to minor minerals and vitamins, most of which are needed in small amounts. No qualified expert would recommend that supplements be used as a substitute for the consumption of good food. If supplements help improve nutrition, they do so by supplementing the food, not by replacing it.

The formulation of a "nutritional insurance" supplement is not easy, and it is a matter of judgment just which of the manageable nutrients are most likely to be deficient in the diets of the general population and what amounts of each should be supplied.

One of the most widely used supplements designed to protect the public against deficiencies, the name of which has almost become a household word, now contains nine vitamins to be taken each day in the following amounts: vitamin A, 5,000 units; vitamin D, 400 units; vitamin B_1, 2 mg; vitamin B_2 (riboflavin), 2.5 mg; vitamin C, 50 mg; vitamin B_6, 1 mg; vitamin B_{12}, 1 mcg; niacinamide, 20 mg; pantothenic acid, 1 mg. This is representative of widely used supplements and can serve as a basis of our discussion.

The amounts of the vitamins included are related to responsible estimates of the desirable amounts for human consumption as follows: vitamin A, 100 percent; vitamin D, 100 percent; vitamin

B_1, 167 percent; vitamin B_2, 167 percent; vitamin C, 111 percent; vitamin B_6, 50 percent; vitamin B_{12}, 33 percent; niacinamide, 133 percent; pantothenic acid, 10 percent. It will be noted that in this formula the historical "favorites," thiamin, riboflavin and niacin which are put into "enriched" flour and bread are provided in generous amounts, whereas such important vitamins as vitamin B_6 and vitamin B_{12} and pantothenic acid are furnished in much smaller amounts. Furthermore, five vitamin-like substances—choline, vitamin E, vitamin K, biotin and folic acid—are left out entirely. For each of these omissions there is a separate but not necessarily adequate reason. Choline is not quite a typical vitamin and is needed in relatively large amounts—about one gram per day; vitamin E is relatively expensive; vitamin K is expensive and often readily produced by intestinal bacteria as is also biotin; folic acid inclusion at appropriate levels has been banned by FDA regulations. All of these five missing vitamins are, however, nutritional essentials, and if one were scientifically formulating a supplement for nutritional insurance the inclusion of each would at least be considered. If regulations prohibit the sale of a good nutritional insurance then perhaps something should be done about the regulations.

The status of vitamin C is special. Convincing evidence has come to light in recent years that young guinea pigs need for good health and development at least 100 times as much vitamin C as they need to protect them from scurvy. Accumulating evidence indicates that human beings may respond similarly. Good nutritional insurance should include far more ascorbic acid than is provided by the popular brand under discussion. (See References 1-5, Chapter 3.)

This supplement is subject to the most severe criticism as a nutritional insurance supplement because it tacitly *assumes* that the only dietary deficiencies are *vitamin* deficiencies. This assumption may be far from valid. No consideration is given to minerals or trace minerals.

One widely advertised preparation recognizes one mineral deficiency, that of iron, and contains seven vitamins and iron. This formulation assumes that other vitamins and other trace minerals not included are inconsequential or the danger of their deficiency is negligible.

In this connection it seems desirable to emphasize again that teamwork among *all* the nutrients is essential. If a person (or an experimental animal) were actually restricted to seven vitamins he would surely die because as far as vitamins are concerned this is an incomplete team. If one were forced to live on iron as the only trace element, he wouldn't live.

If a deficiency were to exist with respect to *one* of the obscure nutrients, *assuming it to be an essential nutrient*, serious damage might result comparable to the damage resulting from ten simultaneous deficiencies. If the metabolic machinery weakens or breaks down, the result is disastrous whether the impairment is due to the defectiveness of one cog or ten cogs.

Nutritional insurance cannot be perfect, but if it is to be used it should be as comprehensive as is feasible. I have never given a great deal of credence to the idea that mice start fires by chewing matches; in spite of my skepticism on this point, however, my house is insured against fire even if it should start in that way. No prudent, well-informed person will buy nutritional insurance that leaves out some contingencies if he can get at a comparable price more complete coverage.

While I have never been in the vitamin business and have never derived profit from any vitamin or supplement formulation, I presently suggest the following vitamin formulation and mineral formulation to be used on a daily basis by those who need insurance. These formulations are subject to change when new information becomes available. No infallibility is claimed.

*Suggested Vitamin Formulation for Nutritional Insurance:**

Vitamin A	7,500 units
Vitamin D	400 units
Vitamin E	40 units
Vitamin K (Menadione)	2 mg
Ascorbic Acid	250 mg

*These suggested vitamin and mineral supplements, designed primarily for adults, can be used without change for teenagers as well. For younger children the amounts can be halved and for very young children the amounts in each case can be diminished to one third of the suggested amounts for adults. For young children who consume mostly milk the iron supplement for adults would probably not be too high. Knowledge regarding the needs at different ages is limited so that hair-splitting discriminations cannot safely be made.

Thiamin	2 mg
Riboflavin	2 mg
Vitamin B$_6$	3 mg
Vitamin B$_{12}$	9 mcg
Niacinamide	20 mg
Pantothenic Acid	15 mg
Biotin	0.3 mg
*Folic Acid	0.4 mg
†Choline	250 mg
†Inositol	250 mg
†P-aminobenzoic acid	30 mg
†Rutin	200 mg

Suggested Mineral Formulation for Nutritional Insurance: ‡

Calcium	250 mg
Phosphate	750 mg (equivalent to 250 mg phosphorous)
Magnesium	200 mg
Iron	15 mg
Zinc	15 mg
Copper	2 mg
Iodine	0.15 mg
§Manganese	5 mg
§Molybdenum	0.1 mg
§Chromium	1.0 mg
§Selenium	0.02 mg
§Cobalt	0.1 mg

Though the *precise* levels to be recommended in the preceding tables are not determinable, the quantitative aspects of these suggested recommendations are nevertheless *all important*. For ex-

*More than the specified amount (about 2 mg) would be recommended if it were not for conflicting FDA regulations.

†These items may have to be excluded if the FDA regulations will not permit their use. Such restriction is, in my opinion, premature and unwise.

‡See footnote, page 75.

§The use of these items may be restricted by the Food and Drug Administration. There is also evidence that tin, nickel and vanadium are needed in traces, but since there is probably a remote chance that people will be deficient in these, they are not listed. Their use is banned by the Food and Drug Administration. Fluoride is also a needed trace mineral but is obtained naturally and in fluoridated water supplies.

ample, one could get *some* of every item in the two lists very simply by consuming a *small morsel* of almost any good food—egg, milk, meat, fish, oyster, mushroom. However, the amount ingested would be entirely negligible unless the food is eaten in quantity. If not, the result would be essentially the same as if nothing had been ingested. This in essence is what happens when one seeks to supplement his diet with a tablet of brewer's yeast or a little wheat germ, alfalfa meal, or "royal jelly." It would take *several ounces* of any of these products daily to yield anything approaching the amount cited in our suggestions. None of these or other similar products or combinations thereof could yield, at any acceptable level, a well-balanced supplement. Carrots, liver, and yellow vegetables are relatively rich sources of vitamin A, but comparable rich natural sources of other vitamins, minerals or amino acids are not to be found.

The vitamin supplement formula and the mineral supplementation formula listed above make no provision for insurance against amino acid deficiencies. To care for this one must, in general, depend on adequate amounts of good protein in one's food. If there are deficiencies in digestion or if such deficiencies are suspected, it may be desirable to recommend the consumption of well-balanced amino acid mixtures which are sometimes available, but expensive. Amino acids are required in too large amounts for them to be included in ordinary supplements.

It should also be noted that the vitamin supplement, as formulated, makes no provision for those who, because of heart or other ailments (or threats of such ailments) or for any other reason, require or desire extra high levels of vitamin A, vitamin E, ascorbic acid, niacinamide or other vitamin. The supplement as formulated is for general, not special, use, and this fact will be reflected by its lower cost. Those who for special reasons may wish to supplement their diets further with additional vitamins or with glutamine, or amino acids will be well advised to use the basic supplement formulated above for general insurance.

How effective would the supplements as formulated be if taken faithfully, and how much insurance would they provide? *No one knows.* On paper and in the light of what we presently know about human nutrition, these supplements should provide valuable insurance, but how valuable this would be it is impossible to know without careful experiments. Much less do we know how much benefit could be derived by administering supposedly improved modifications of these supplements.

There seems to be no good reason why we need to remain in ignorance regarding the usefulness of a proposed supplement. If one group of individuals were given the proposed supplement and a comparable group was given placebos, and if the health of each member in the study were monitored by periodic objective bio-chemical and other measurements, it should be possible in a rela-tively short time to see whether or not the supplement conferred benefit. The conclusiveness of this experiment would hinge in part upon the ability of the experimenters, using modern tech-nology and common sense, to monitor people's health without depending on subjective judgments such as those obtained by asking each individual subject periodically, "How do you feel today"? Answers to this and similar questions might be of some value if the experiment were done on a double-blind basis, but otherwise would be of little value.

What other kinds of supplements can there be beside these de-signed for insurance purposes? There might be desirable supple-ments suitable for people with different types of chronic maladies. However, since the experts on disease (the physicians) and nutri-tional experts have never joined hands to deal with the basic problems, there are no supplements that I could suggest for specific diseased conditions. "Therapeutic" formulas usually contain con-siderably more of certain vitamins, but what they are "therapeutic" for remains something of a mystery.

During the past few years there has developed what is called the "orthomolecular" approach particularly to mental disease; this involves nutritional supplementation. In the book *Orthomolecular Psychiatry*, Pauling and Hawkins, editors, there is presented some of the material in this field. I would find it difficult, and I am sure many of my physician-readers would also, to evaluate critically all the clinical findings.

I feel very strongly, however, that the principle behind this approach is sound and unassailable. The essential idea is to use in combatting mental disease those substances which are naturally in the brain rather than depending on foreign agents which accidentally may seem to confer benefit. In other words, the fundamental idea is *to bring the brain biochemistry back to normal.*

In order to accomplish this purpose, rather massive doses of some of the vitamins have been used with seeming effectiveness. For reasons which we do not fully understand, probably related to digestion, absorption and transport, some vitamins become effective in some individuals only when the intake is very high. This whole subject badly needs to be explored further, and the effectiveness of such treatment needs to be investigated and evaluated, especially when it is combined with a good general nutritional supplementation.

This vast subject is too large to be dealt with more fully in this chapter.

About forty years ago I conceived the idea that alcoholism is probably a genetotrophic disease. This means that the susceptible victims probably have unusual nutritional demands which are not easily met; if these demands can be met by using supplements, then the victim's condition should improve. Following this lead and based on extensive animal experimentation, I suggested the use of various supplements somewhat similar to those listed above. However, in the case of alcoholics I suggested that several daily quotas of vitamins should be taken each day on the suspicion that some of the vitamins were needed by these individuals in much larger than the usual amounts. The alcoholics were also advised how to eat rationally and to include in their diet a good complement of unsaturated fat acids in the form of salad oil. While there have been no adequate controlled experiments[3] to test the validity of the application of the basic genetotrophic idea, thousands of alcoholics have seemingly received benefit, and in a large number of cases the results have been most dramatic. On top of these, there have been many individuals who seemingly have been benefited remarkably by another supplement, glutamine. A nutritional supplement designed to combat alcoholism and protect against it should include glutamine in substantial amounts, probably two grams per day in divided doses.

The rationale behind the use of such supplements for alcoholism is relatively simple. The mechanisms in the brain which regulate the desire for food, for water, for sugar, and probably other items need complete and adequate nourishment and can go awry when this nourishment is deficient *in any way*. In the case of an alcoholic, it is impossible to get good nutrition to the brain while consuming alcohol in quantity. Hence an alcoholic's brain is liable to become deficient in the nutrients that are limiting factors in his general nutrition. Furthermore, at higher levels of concentration alcohol is definitely poisonous and can help bring about metabolic derangement. Whatever the theory behind the phenomenon is, alcoholics *invariably* cultivate a perverted appetite. In extreme cases they lose all desire for food; the sight or smell of it becomes nauseating. Instead, they have an insatiable appetite for alcohol.

It is high time, I think, that medical scientists look carefully into the biochemical and nutritional factors involved in alcoholism, and cease to fall back on blaming it all onto vague psychological factors which are difficult to spot or to deal with. This condition, alcoholism, which affects severely about 9 million people in the United States and less severely many millions more, is one in which suitable supplements judiciously used can probably bring tremendous benefit. Good nutrition, if consistently received, can definitely prevent alcoholism. It usually takes several years of flagrant nutritional abuse to bring about full-blown alcoholism.

In light of our discussion of biochemical individuality it is reasonable to assume that certain individuals in a large population will have what appear to be bizarre nutritional needs and deficiencies. The "typical" individual has some needs that are "far from average."[4] Because of these deficiencies some individuals may be afflicted with all sorts of unexpected and unexplained disorders.[5] Probably some rare individuals would be benefited if zinc alone were used as a supplement; others might be greatly benefited by lysine alone, pantothenic acid alone, or any other single nutrient. Others might be benefited by supplements containing two or three or more nutrients if the selection happened to meet the individual's need. In the light of these considerations it is dangerous to pooh-pooh the observation of a patient who claims to be benefited by a specific nutrient or a specific supplement, even though the supplement was poorly conceived and compounded. It is also dangerous to deny categorically that the topical administration of a vitamin or a supplement can bring benefit. Iodine painted on one's big toe will cure the endemic goiter which is due to lack of iodine.

Nutritional supplements have never been a favorite part of the armamentarium of most physicians, and changes will not come overnight. Assuming the role of a prophet, I will predict that in years to come supplements will be used more and more and with greater intelligence. Especially will they have an appeal if automated and computerized techniques are developed so that the metabolic profiles of individuals can be determined. These profiles, even if circumscribed, may at least give some hints as to what the peculiar needs of individuals are.

Hyperalimentation which involves parenteral feeding is related to the use of nutritional supplements.[6,7] When "intravenous feeding" has been practiced in decades past, it involved the administration of glucose in saline solution. This, of course, is feeding only in a very restricted sense; it furnishes only the necessary fuel and none of the nonfuel nutrients needed to build and maintain the metabolic machinery in cells. Glucose feeding can be justified as an emergency measure on the grounds that the individual's tissues are probably intact and have reserves to take care of short-term deprivations.

Hyperalimentation, on the other hand, involves administration of far more complete nutrition. This procedure, from the standpoint of nutritional expertise, has been developed and exploited only in a limited way.

This brings to mind the fact that physicians have at their disposal methods of administration of nutrients that are not available to nutritionists or other nonphysicians—administration by injection. In case a patient is suffering from deficiency caused wholly or in part by defective digestion, absorption or transport (these may be relatively common), the physician can administer the nutrients in question in any way he sees fit. Nonphysicians do not have this option. This is one of the many reasons why nutritional therapy should be supervised by physicians.

I should like to see the procedure of hyperalimentation further developed and its use extended. I believe that untold benefit might accrue if this procedure, when refined, were used routinely on all psychiatric patients before drug or shock treatment is instituted.

There is excellent reason for thinking that the difficulties might be made to vanish by this means. This hope is fostered by the assumption that a mentally ill person is really ill, and that something in his brain is not functioning normally. If this is true, it is highly probable that the environment (rather than the heredity) of the brain cells is defective. The nutritional environment certainly needs scrutiny, and it probably needs modification and improvement. Hyperalimentation might easily accomplish the desired end because it might furnish the brain cells directly the wherewithal to rebuild themselves.

REFERENCES

1. Heinz, H.J.: Nutritional illiteracy. Newspaper article in *New York Times*, January 14, 1972.
2. One third of a nation: A report on young men found unqualified for military service. Compiled by the President's Task Force on Manpower. January 1, 1964.
3. Trulson, M.F., Fleming, R.F., and Stare, F.J.: Vitamin medication in alcoholism. *J.A.M.A., 155*:114, 1954.
4. Burton, B.T. (Ed.): *Heinz Handbook on Nutrition.* New York, McGraw, 1959, p. 137.
5. Alverez, W.C.: *Practical Leads to Puzzling Diagnoses.* Philadelphia, Lippincott, 1958.
6. Dudrick, S.J., and Ruberg, R.L.: Principles and practice of parenteral nutrition. *Gastroenterology, 61*:901, 1971.
7. Dudrick, S.J., and Copeland, E.M.: Parenteral hyperalimentation. In Nyhus, L.M. (Ed.): *Surgery Annual.* New York, Appleton, 1973.

CHAPTER 10

THE CONTAMINATION
OR POLLUTION OF
NUTRITIONAL ENVIRONMENTS

WE NEED to be concerned about the contamination or pollution of our air, water and food because our external environment immediately becomes a part of the internal environment of our cells and tissues. Pollution in the external environment spells pollution of the internal environment.

The term *contaminants* denotes all those substances which are foreign to an ideal environment regardless of how harmless or how damaging they may be. I avoid using the word *pollutants* as equivalent to *contaminants* because I do not wish to prejudge and imply that what is foreign necessarily does serious damage. A pollutant *spoils* the environment, and we need to consider the possibility, at least, that a contaminant may do no appreciable harm.

Whether a contaminant does appreciable harm depends on its nature and on the quantity present. The quantitative aspects of contamination and pollution are all-important, as are the quantitative aspects of nutrition. It is meaningless to say, "I had some vitamin A in my dinner today," just as it is meaningless to say, "Our available air contains sulfur dioxide, hydrogen sulfide, ammonia and carbon monoxide." We must know something about the amounts involved if we are to make an intelligent remark or participate in an intelligent discussion about either nutrition or pollution.

An illustration should make clear the crucial importance of appreciating the quantitative aspects of contamination or pollution. Suppose a liter sample of air were stated to contain about 500 billion molecules each of sulfur dioxide and hydrogen sulfide, also 15 trillion molecules of ammonia, and 250 trillion molecules of carbon monoxide. This would suggest that we are describing badly polluted air. Such a conclusion would, however, reveal a complete lack of perspective brought about by the distortion of the *quantitative aspects* by expressing the amounts present in unsuitable units (numbers of molecules).

Expressed in proper terms, the amounts of sulfur dioxide, hydrogen sulfide, ammonia and carbon monoxide present in the sample of air under discussion are, respectively: 0.02 pp. billion, 0.02 pp. billion, 0.6 pp. billion, and 0.01 pp. million. This air would probably be freer from these contaminants than any air ever breathed by a human being![1] Traces of these and other contaminants are always present in the atmosphere and always will be as long as there are volcanoes, sulfur springs, forest fires (or other open fires), thunderstorms and decaying matter. Even in the relatively pure air of coastal cities like San Diego and San Francisco, the four contaminants we have listed are commonly present in amounts at least 100 times as great as in the sample of air we used in our illustration.[2]

The importance of looking at pollution problems *with perspective and with due regard for the quantitative aspects* cannot be exaggerated.

No argument can be made that it is good to have sulfur dioxide, hydrogen sulfide, ammonia, carbon monoxide, oxides of nitrogen, etc. in the air we breathe, but if the levels are very low (we can hardly remedy the situation) our bodies have ways of taking care of the trace amounts. When the levels become as high as they do in many cities, contamination may be an entirely different matter. In this case, levels of contaminants should be monitored and judged by experts who know about the quantities that can readily be tolerated. Our air environment, like our climatic environment and our food environment, is never perfect, just tolerable in varying degrees.

Scare headlines, uncritical and inexpert emotional discussions of air pollution are unproductive and do not contribute to the understanding or to the solution of the problems.[3] That people are often able to tolerate air contaminants with little damage is indicated by the fact that members of my profession, chemists, often work in contaminated atmospheres and yet do not have to pay higher life insurance premiums because of this fact. Among my chemist friends and acquaintances have been one who is hale and hearty and past ninety, one who worked daily in his chemical laboratory until his death at the age of eighty-nine, and another who was active in the laboratory until he was nearly 100 years of age. I am not advocating having contaminated air in chemical laboratories, but I do urge that the problem of air pollution be viewed realistically and in perspective, considering all the facts. The dangers of air pollution do not look as bleak as they would if chemists were in the habit of dying off at an early age.

It is not my purpose in this chapter to deal with the contamination of our internal environments in anything approaching an exhaustive manner. Such contamination comes from the air we breathe, the water we drink, and from whatever we consume. The contaminants are numerous and have many origins. There are many reliable sources of information *of a quantitative nature* to be found in books and articles. All I can hope to do is to cite some of the more salient facts and to present them in reasonable perspective.

One of the occasions for food contamination by foreign chemicals is our continual combat against our insect and other enemies. When we poison them we are in danger of poisoning ourselves unless we exercise great care. Because of the biochemical unity in nature, chemicals that are poisonous to one species are very likely to be more or less poisonous for others. Because of its wide use in insect control and the fact that it is not easily destroyed in nature, DDT has gained notoriety in the public mind. Chemists have learned to detect extremely tiny amounts of this substance. This may be regarded as a tribute to the prowess of chemists; the fact that DDT can be detected so widely does not prove that it is at dangerous levels. It is of course dangerous only when the amounts present in the total environment reach levels that cannot be readily tolerated by us or the birds and other animals we care about. Investigations directed toward finding substitute chemical insecticides which do not persist in nature so long are very much in order.

When it was discovered nearly fifty years ago that tetraethyl lead, when added to gasoline, greatly improved its anti-knock properties, this was considered a triumph. Now we realize that its use in gasoline has widely disseminated a dangerous poison and that we must seek by all feasible means to avoid the dangerous consequences. How dangerous this poison is to human life under present or anticipated conditions is a question we will not discuss in detail. Lead is a slow acting poison, but it is also cumulative. The *amounts* which people may get is a crucial question. An interesting sidelight is the fact, demonstrated with guinea pigs,[4] that adequate intake of ascorbic acid has a strong protective effect in preventing lead poisoning.

Because foods have to be stored, packaged, shipped and kept in condition to sell, and also because it is desirable for foods to be attractive in appearance and taste, a very large number of additives are permitted by the Food and Drug Administration to be added to food. Hundreds of these additives are permitted, many of them for highly technical reasons associated with food production.

Some estimates are to the effect that we commonly consume about three pounds of these nonnutritive additives per capita per year. Certainly most of these substances are relatively harmless at the levels used. Possibly they are no more dangerous than the traces of hydrogen sulfide, sulfur dioxide, ammonia, and carbon monoxide commonly present in "pure" air. Some of the allowed additives may be at dangerous levels, but this is certainly debatable, and my own impression is that the Food and Drug Administration handles these problems in a relatively satisfactory manner. Always the *amounts* involved must be considered.

These chemical additives are used for inhibiting the development of molds, for stabilizing emulsions, for insect repellants, emulsifiers, anti-oxidants, fruit flavors, tenderizers, coloring agents, etc. The amounts of these chemical agents consumed *per year* may give a distorted picture unless we consider some other comparable figures on a *yearly* basis. For comparison, while we may consume three pounds in the aggregate of hundreds of nonnutritive chemicals in a year, we take from the air, which in the popular mind is almost weightless, well over 500 *pounds* of oxygen each year. While each of us is said to eat a peck of dirt during a lifetime, this is neither a very alarming nor a very important observation.

The danger derived from having foreign substances in food is determined by their nature and the *amount* present. This idea is strongly supported by well-authenticated facts regarding the presence of toxicants in practically all common natural foods.[5] Usually in the foods we commonly consume these toxicants are present in such small amounts that they cause no worry, but they are present *in traces* in potatoes, sweet potatoes, cabbages, carrots, tomatoes, fruits, wheat, rice, oats, corn, buckwheat, beans, peas, peanuts, almonds and other nuts, cheese, eggs, fish, shellfish, etc., and in the flesh and milk of animals that forage on plants. Most often the toxicants found in plants are complicated organic substances belonging among the glycosides and alkaloids. Some are more complicated. Sometimes plants carry poisonous amounts of trace elements such as selenium and molybdenum.

That we human beings must select our foods in such a way as to avoid those which carry larger amounts of toxicants is evident when we consider the undesirability of consuming meals containing baked castor beans, tobacco greens, oleander salad or mushrooms of the wrong varieties. Even coffee beans, because of their caffeine content, would not contribute to a wholesome meal. Improperly stored or moldy foods often carry toxicants in relatively unsafe amounts. Since natural foods contain traces of undesirable chemicals, and sometimes these chemicals may be present in more than perfectly safe amounts, it is probably desirable *for this reason* not to concentrate on the consumption of one food or of a very few foods. This is, then, another reason for diversification in the selection of foods. We are more likely to tolerate trace amounts of numerous toxicants than we are to tolerate relatively larger amounts of a few.

It is human nature for people, when things appear to go wrong, to try to find someone else or something outside themselves to blame. When a person's health is not the best, one way to rationalize is to suppose that somebody has been contaminating his or her food. In some cases, of course, this suspicion may be justified.

I would like, however, to call attention to the self-pollution which is commonly practiced. Ray Lyman Wilbur, a physician who was President of Stanford University when I was a professor in a neighboring university, said

> Most people have but little idea how to care for their bodies or how to use their brains and be well and happy. Millions of them keep themselves under the partial influence of caffeine, alcohol, nicotine, aspirin, and other drugs a good deal of the time. From childhood they never play fair with the finest machine on earth. The doctors themselves are not always good examples, and many of them care for their automobiles better than they do for themselves.[6]

In his little "sermon" Dr. Wilbur mentioned, not necessarily in the order of their importance, the outstanding contaminants of our internal environment which we deliberately introduce: *Caffeine, alcohol, nicotine, aspirin,* and *other drugs.* These are things that people take into their systems because they like them or their effects. Several of them are habit forming, and some, of course, are addictive.

There is no way of measuring just how much harmful (or beneficial) effects caffeine has on human beings. The lethal dose of caffeine (L.D.$_{50}$) for several animals is about 200 mg/kg, while the *average* per capita consumption in the United States of America is calculated to be about 8 mg/kg per day.[1] Since babies, children and many adults get little or none, it is obvious that some individuals get several times the average amount. In our laboratories we recently tried to feed rats a diet containing caffeine at the level, per calorie, of average human consumption. Shortly they began to chew their feet (a characteristic symptom of caffeine toxicity), and we had to change the diet to one that contained instant decaffeinated coffee instead of instant coffee. These considerations suggest that contamination of one's internal environments with caffeine can be far from negligible, especially when it is recognized that some individuals are far above others in their susceptibility to "poisoning" by caffeine.

Alcohol is, of course, a familiar contaminant of our internal environment; if one is very moderate in its consumption, according to usual standards, (a 1½ oz. jigger of distilled liquor per day), he gets about sixteen grams of alcohol per day. If this were introduced into the blood at one time, this would yield about five times the concentration known to be associated with toxic effects (intoxication). Since some individuals are immoderate in their alcohol consumption and some are highly susceptible to its toxic effects, it is not surprising that about 9 million people in the United States are so badly poisoned that their appetite mechanisms are seriously deranged.

Nicotine contamination of our internal environment can be very harmful in spite of the fact that the amounts ingested are relatively small. Nicotine is a powerful poison (active in very small amounts) and for some is addictive. People pollute their internal environment with nicotine because they like its immediate effects, and no nicotineless smoke or chew is an effective substitute. This is not to say or suggest that the harmfulness of smoking or chewing tobacco is due to nicotine alone.

The contamination of one's internal environment with "aspirin and other drugs" is a part of a very large problem. It is not easy to place the blame, but in our culture (not to say that it is absent in others) there is a strong tendency to say to ourselves, in effect, "If something goes wrong, *try contaminating the internal environment and see if it doesn't help.*"

If one has a little private pain, headache or distress after a heavy meal, he seeks to find some appropriate contaminant which will give relief. If one gets sleepy when he or she doesn't want to, or if one is wakeful when wanting to go to sleep, the accepted recourse is to reach for something (a contaminant) which can help. If a person wants to eat less, he would like to find something he could take to reduce his appetite; if he wants to eat more (this is rarer) he would like to find a contaminant that when taken would stimulate his appetite. If a person's sex urge is low or waning, he or she would like to reach for a contaminant that would remedy the situation. If one is not as bright intellectually as he desires, he may yearn for a "small pill" that will pull him through the coming examination.

Prevention of bad breath, of sour stomach, of sunburn, of that "tired feeling," of mental depression, of lack of stamina, of insect bites and what not, call for the same general remedy: Reach for a pill that will overcome the trouble.

This policy has become axiomatic, and axioms are dangerous. This axiom is like the one we too often accept, "Avoid physical exertion at all costs. Get something (a labor-saving device) or somebody else to do it for you."

If people were to go to doctors for help in finding the right medicine, the situation would be greatly improved. But the axiomatic principle "Reach for something" is still open to question.

It seems to me that the wide acceptance of the idea that the way to overcome difficulties is to find some external agent that will bring relief is basic to the widespread tendency of young people to "try" marijuana, LSD, amphetamines, pep pills, heroin or anything else that gives promise of bringing happiness even though in an unreal dream world.

Passing laws and trying to enforce them is a direct way to attack the drug problem, but a more effective and lasting remedy may lie in training young people, from childhood, to appreciate on a scientific basis how important our internal environments are and how the contamination and pollution of these environments is always subject to dangerous (and perhaps fatal) consequences.

REFERENCES

1. Robbins, E., and Robbins, R.C.: Emissions concentrations and fate of gaseous atmospheric pollutants. In Strauss, W. (Ed.): *Air Pollution Control II.* New York, Wiley, 1972.
2. Babcock, L.A.: A combined pollution index for measurement of total air pollution. *J. A.P.C.A. 20:653,* 1970.
3. Standen, A. (Ed.): *Encyclopedia of Chemical Technology,* 2nd ed. New York, Wiley, 1963, Vol. X.
4. Pilleman, L., et al.: Chronic lead poisoning. *Am. J. Med. Sci. 200:322,* 1940.
5. *Naturally Occurring Toxicants in Foods.* National Academy of Sciences-National Research Council Publication 1354. Washington, D.C. 1966.
6. Gray, George W.: *Advancing Front of Medicine.* New York, McGraw, 1941, p. 394.
7. Deuchmann, W.B., and Gerarde, H.W.: *Symptomatology and Therapy of Toxicological Emergencies.* New York, Acad Pr, 1964.

CHAPTER 11

WHAT IS NOT KNOWN ABOUT CLINICAL NUTRITION

THE LISTING of the things we do not know about nutrition may be more arduous than listing what we do know.

The names of the chemical substances we must get nutritionally from our environment may justifiably be considered the "nutritional alphabet," because nutrition, if it is to be approached intelligently, must be dealt with in terms of these substances. We do not yet know the complete "nutritional alphabet." Furthermore, if the principle of teamwork holds, it is extremely important that we consider all members of the team. One weak link in the chain of our knowledge can be disastrous. In a sense all scientific nutrition must suffer at least a limp until the alphabet is complete.

The status of lipoic acid in this regard is uncertain. This substance independently discovered and synthesized in our laboratory has all the earmarks of a B vitamin *except* that it appears that it can be made endogenously by mammals. My colleague, Dr. Lester Reed, has isolated multienzyme complexes in which lipoic acid is an essential unit. One of these units which is a representative part of the total metabolic machinery of cells contains forty-two enzyme molecules of three different sorts, all bound together in a specific known geometrical pattern. One sort contains thiamin (vitamin B_1); another sort contains riboflavin (vitamin B_2), and the third kind contains lipoic acid. The whole complex is necessary to bring about the dehydrogenation of pyruvate. When the complex is broken down to its constituent enzymes, it loses its activity, but the activity is restored when the complex is allowed to reconstitute itself.[1]

This information with respect to lipoic acid is given to show that knowledge regarding its functioning is relatively far advanced, and there is no doubt whatever about its vital role in metabolism.

Though most authorities in the field of nutrition would probably categorically deny that lipoic acid is essential for the nutrition of mammals or fowls, there are some observations which make me wonder. In our laboratories we observed that it promoted the growth of young rats when included in the diet.[2] Mardones has found that its inclusion in the diet decreases the appetite of rats for alcohol.[3] Investigators in other laboratories failed to confirm that it is an essential nutrient. The only explanation we can offer is that under our experimental conditions, using a particular strain (and group) of rats, it functioned in a manner not duplicated elsewhere.

Also in our laboratory it was found under specified conditions to stimulate in a clear-cut way the growth of baby chicks. Subsequently we have repeated the experiment and have obtained equally clear-cut negative results. Even more puzzling is the fact that in the Du Pont Laboratories they have had a similar experience. At one time they have obtained statistically significant positive responses with chicks; they have also obtained results that are clearly negative.

The best summary of the situation which I can give is as follows: lipoic acid without question acts in metabolism like a B vitamin, but appears to be made endogenously at least under many circumstances. It is probably nonessential nutritionally, but it may be one of the "desirables" we have referred to in an earlier discussion.

Another substance with a somewhat uncertain status is inositol. It is not known to act in catalytic systems like a B vitamin, but years ago it was found when given nutritionally to prevent alopecia in mice. The earliest observation regarding its nutritional efficacy was made in connection with yeast. It is definitely a yeast nutrient.

My judgment is that it probably can be made endogenously in mammals under ordinary conditions but that animals may thrive better under some circumstances when it is provided by the environment. Perhaps it is one of the "desirables."

Further evidence that the nutritional alphabet is not completely known is the fact that animals on diets of known composition (containing all the presently known alphabet members) do not breed well. It is true that Schultze[4] has raised experimental animals on synthetic diets through three generations, but there was a downhill trend on the part of the animals' vigor and their reproductive record as the program was continued. It has long been observed in our laboratories (though not tested rigorously in experiments) that experimental animals breed better when their chow diets are supplemented with fresh vegetables. What is present in fresh vegetables to improve the diet is unknown. We have recently obtained fresh objective evidence in our laboratories that fresh vegetables contain some nutritional unknown or unknowns not hitherto recognized.

A protracted and perhaps highly significant investigation initiated at the Rockefeller Institute (now Rockefeller University) suggests that there may be a number of "unknowns" in nutrition yet to be explored. Schneider has discovered and concentrated to a high degree a substance found in many foods which, when added to the diet of mice (200 to 400 parts per billion), will protect them from salmonella infection.[5] How this nutritional substance is related to others which may exist and may help protect human beings from infection is unknown.

Still another reason for thinking that there are nutritional unknowns (missing alphabet members) is the fact that when somatic cells are grown in tissue culture one is invariably confronted with the necessity of adding to the culture medium some undefined material like embryonic tissue extract or blood serum. If all the alphabet members were known, it should be possible to culture various human cells at will without resorting to the use of mixtures of unknown compositions. Among the still unrecognized nutrients may be such trace elements as tin, vanadium, arsenic or others.

This brings us to the discussion of another area where "unknowns" are unquestionably involved. A pertinent question is: What substances are involved in intercellular symbiosis? Glutamine, for example, must be produced by certain cells in our bodies and furnished to other cells which cannot live without a source outside themselves. What other such substances exist? It seems probable that lipoic acid and inositol belong in this category, and there are probably others, possibly many of them. If so, they are cell nutrients in a very real sense.

Among the organic nutrients already known, there are several the functions of which are relatively well understood. This is true in general of the B vitamins which play catalytic roles in numerous enzyme systems. Regarding certain other organic nutrients, however, we are mostly in the dark.

The functioning of vitamin A in connection with the building of visual pigments has been known for decades. However, this is only one function of this vitamin as is shown by the fact that vitamin A acid, while not effective as a precursor of visual pigments, can perform other functions which make possible the life and reproduction of experimental animals. What these other functions are is unknown. A recent study has come to my attention indicating that vitamin A acid can prevent skin cancers in mice. The health of all epithelial tissue is thought to depend on an adequate supply of vitamin A, but why, we do not know.[6]

The functions of vitamin C are also obscure. It is known chemically to be an antioxidant, but its biological effect is not duplicated by other antioxidants. It is known to be involved in some obscure way in the building of hydroxyproline and hydroxylysine into collagen, but again this fails to explain its role satisfactorily. Does it have antiviral activity; if so, how and just what effects does it have on "colds?" Numerous people, including many scientists and physicians, are thoroughly convinced, on the basis of personal experience, that it often acts as a preventative and curative agent.

One of the basic reasons why we need to know about the functions of vitamins A and C is because we need light on the problem of how there can possibly be such wide variation from individual to individual in the apparent needs for these vitamins. To say that some guinea pigs seem to need twenty times as much vitamin C as others for best performance is to state the case very conservatively. It would be difficult also to exaggerate the differences we have found in the apparent vitamin A needs of different individual rats. We had groups of weanling rats on four different levels of vitamin A intake: 0, 1, 4 and 64 units per day per rat respectively. Some rats at the lower levels of intake gained very little weight, and several died within a few weeks. In spite of this, there were relatively healthy survivors; after 110 days on these diets we were able to select from each of the four groups receiving from 0 to 64 units per day per rat, individual animals which were similarly healthy and well developed. From the standpoint of vigor and appearance these selected animals from the four groups could not be distinguished from each other. If these surviving animals alone were considered, one would be tempted to conclude that for 110 days young rats do not need vitamin A. This was not an experiment which encompassed the lifetime of the rats, it is true, but during the time from youth to maturity the apparent needs were extraordinarily diverse. How can this possibly be? If we knew more adequately the functions of vitamin A and ascorbic acid we might be able to make sense out of these observations. As they stand, such observations appear so outlandish that the more traditionally oriented nutritionists tend to look the other way.

The functions of the other "fat soluble" vitamins (other than the visual functions of vitamin A), vitamin D, vitamin E, vitamin K, are likewise obscure, although good progress has recently been made with respect to the D vitamins.[7]

I well remember when it was discovered that experimental rats require fat in their diet. It was observed that without fat in the diet, tail lesions developed. Some nutritionists apparently tended to deduce that since human beings typically have no tails, this observation is of little human interest. For decades the question of the human need for fat (or for particular unsaturated fat acids) was in doubt. The functioning of these fat acids is still obscure, and whether and to what extent fat is needed or is desirable in human and animal diets badly needs further exploration.

One of the basic areas of ignorance in the nutritional field has to do with self-selection of food. While some nutritionists deny that self-selection plays any important role, there are certain facts which suggest strongly the idea that self-selection on the part of individuals may play a large role in helping them get what they need and avoiding what is deleterious, and that by proper attention this role can be increased.

One fact related to this problem is undeniable. Healthy people and healthy animals, especially those living active lives, *often* possess internal regulating mechanisms which cause them to eat (without study, deliberation or counting calories) almost *exactly* the right amount of food to take care of their metabolic needs. The fact that there are people who have difficulties in this area in no way denies the existence of those who have no difficulty or very little. If an individual person (and there are many such) eats spontaneously and neither gains nor loses more than five pounds per year, this means that his internal regulating mechanisms work with an error of about

0.3 percent or less. An individual may consume around 1,500 pounds of food in a year, and if his regulatory mechanism were to overshoot the mark, causing him to consume and assimilate 1 percent more than was burned up during the year, this would mean a gain in weight of about fifteen pounds. If this continued for ten years it would mean a gain of 150 pounds. Even the worst regulating mechanism possessed by any of us still makes a very small percentage error. If anyone of us in affluent circumstances were to go into a restaurant *leaving his regulating mechanism entirely behind,* the result would be fatal engorgement. In real life we know that when anyone, no matter how gluttonous or obese, has eaten for awhile, he begins to lose his hunger. We also know that in all cases the internal regulating mechanism is somewhat selective. It tells the individual not to eat the entire contents of the sugar bowl or the salt shaker or to order and consume a pound of butter. Nausea and distaste would stop him. Our regulatory mechanisms in general are at least *somewhat operative and selective,* not only with respect to how much we eat but also as to how much of each food we eat.

The crucial questions are: *How* selective can our mechanisms be and is there any way the performance of these mechanisms can be improved?

A strong hint that our internal regulatory mechanisms may be of substantial help to us is found in the observation that rats can distinguish between a *complete* mixture of essential amino acids and an *incomplete* mixture which is missing one of the essential cogs.[8,9] This is done obviously without their having any knowledge of what an amino acid is.

Do human beings have corresponding mechanisms and are these mechanisms potentially capable of helping us make many discriminating judgments and wise selections? This we do not know, and this is one reason why the question of self-selection has been designated as an area of ignorance.

That this type of "body wisdom" can be cultivated (and probably also made inoperative) is indicated by the old observation made decades ago that well-nourished children by self-selection eat less candy than children who have had poor nutrition. (This has also been confirmed in our laboratory with baby rats.) In the United States we consume on the average about 105 pounds of sugar per capita per year. Some, of course, get far more than their share. According to evidence collected by some medical authorities, this amount is harmful, and we would be far better off with respect to heart disease, for example, if our per capita consumption were a fraction of this amount.[10]

A possible explanation of why we eat so much sugar is that as babies we were forced to get an early start when our formulas consisted of cow's milk sweetened generously with sugar. Over the years the appetite for sugar is cultivated and accentuated by mediocre nutrition. If this idea is valid, and too much sugar is harmful, at least a partial remedy would be to use glucose instead of sucrose (they are not physiologically equivalent) in baby formulas and decrease the amount.

Regardless of one's attitude toward sugar consumption, the general idea that good nutrition should foster "body wisdom" and the building of effective regulatory mechanisms (whatever they are able to do) is hard to attack. The brain cells (or other cells) involved in these mechanisms should fare better if they are well supplied with the essential nutrients. Poor nutrition would be expected to impair "body wisdom," and this in turn could set up a vicious cycle.

Experience in the army and elsewhere has shown that it is quite impractical and unrealistic to expect different individuals to eat identically the same food. When given a selection, different individuals choose very distinctively. If a group is served generously in a uniform way, what they leave on their plates, in spite of social pressures, is far from uniform. Custom and culture has probably tended to make people eat more alike than if they had not been subject to social constraints.

We have made a start in investigating this phenomenon of food choice in young weanling rats which had no previous conditioning with respect to choice of food.[11] We gave each of a group of thirty-nine young rats a "cafeteria selection" for a period of seventeen days and kept a record of the food consumed by each rat. The selections consisted of (1) dried lean meat, (2) butter, (3) sugar, (4) raw carrots, (5) salt mixture, (6) fortified yeast. The thirty-nine animals exhibited about a four-fold range in their consumption of meat, salt and carrots. For butter the range was seven-fold, for sugar seventeen-fold, and for the fortified yeast forty-six-fold! Many studies in our laboratories have shown that even inbred rats exhibit a high degree of biological individuality. In this case, *why* are their appetites so consistently diverse? What do the animals accomplish? Are they exhibiting some kind of "body wisdom," or is it "body foolishness?" Regardless of interpretation the fact remains that they have individual appetites that are highly distinctive and strikingly different. It may be inferred that human beings would also exhibit wide differences in appetites if social influences did not induce them to become more uniform.

If our current nutrition in the United States is lacking in quality, part of the difficulty may lie in the tendency to make children (and adults) eat in a uniform manner and not to encourage them to develop their own body wisdom.

The facts of biochemical individuality make this possibility a real consideration. Each of us needs a distinctive assortment of nutrients (quantitatively speaking). How can we fulfill our own individual needs if we are forced to be uniform? Do we have innate internal mechanisms that can potentially help us? This is a big question to which we do not know the answer.

That such mechanisms exist and actually operate is indicated when we realize that all natural foods contain traces of toxicants which are capable of causing trouble when consumed in sufficient amounts. The existence of wide variance in the responses of individuals to many specific drugs is widely recognized. It therefore seems probable that unusually susceptible individuals might be bothered by concentrations of toxicants that would be of no concern to others. This is probably at least a partial basis of the old saying of the Latin Lucretius, "What is one man's meat is another's poison."

This interpretation may have merit in helping understand why some otherwise "normal" people have special dislikes for certain good foods such as cabbage, spinach, eggplant, string beans or what not. Maybe they are peculiarly susceptible to the toxicants present in these foods. I have known of people becoming severely if not seriously ill from consuming raw turnips or from eating quantities of peanuts. Rejection by vomiting is, of course, one way the body has of ridding itself of objectionable material. Perhaps the toxicants in foods are often responsible for making people "sick to their stomachs." As we have mentioned earlier, one way an individual can help diminish such trouble is to diversify his eating and not eat large amounts of any one food which may carry a toxicant to which he may be peculiarly susceptible.

The vast field of "food allergies" and idiosyncracies is related to our present discussion and is included in the areas of ignorance we have been discussing.[12] There are many postulations, many guesses, many interesting and striking individual experiences, but a basic understanding of the whole problem is for the future. The recognition and consideration of the biochemical individuality involved cannot be escaped.

Having spent a substantial part of my scientific career doing pioneer investigation with respect to two vitamins, pantothenic acid and folic acid, both of which I named, it is natural that my mind is directed toward unanswered questions about these nutrients.

One question in this category is, can ingesting extra pantothenic acid prolong life? The fact that this vitamin is a prominent constituent of "royal jelly" which does, when provided nutritionally, prolong the life of a female honeybee from a few weeks up to several years, suggested an experiment to determine whether extra pantothenic acid would prolong the life of mice.[7] (See Chap. 8, Ref. 31.) It did prolong their life about 19 percent; so now the question is, will it do similarly for human beings? We do not know. No one has ever tried it out.

"Royal jelly" which was for many years the richest known natural source of pantothenic acid, when fed to a bee larva, completely transforms its life. What would otherwise become a sterile worker bee becomes a "queen" which during a long life of several years lays many thousands of fertile eggs. The question stimulated by a recognition of these facts is: "Can pantothenic acid be of value in promoting a better reproductive record in animals and in man?"

Feeding extra pantothenic acid to hens has been found to cause an increased hatchability of their eggs,[13] and feeding extra pantothenic acid to pregnant mice and rats improved their reproductive record by increasing the size of their litters. I would say that the presumption is, especially in view of some of our previous discussions (see Chap. 8, p. 56), that giving extra pantothenic acid to pregnant women would probably improve the quality of their offspring and lessen the incidence of birth deformities and of the birth of mentally retarded babies. This possibility has never been tested. One dean of a medical school in this country has written me (1971) that at present the human reproductive record in the United States is "terrible."

Another question is: "Is pantothenic acid an important factor in the prevention and treatment of alcoholism?" I know of investigators who think it is, but I don't know. It is a matter of conjecture.

I have before me a thirty-two-page booklet entitled, "Arthritis: A Vitamin Deficiency Disease," by Dr. E. Barton-Wright of London, a reputable investigator whom I have known of for many years.[14] The vitamin in question is pantothenic acid, and the author in his concluding discussion says:

"If the author's arguments and interpretation of the data be correct, then it follows that if every individual could be sure of consuming at least 25 to 50 mg of pantothenic acid in his or her daily diet, arthritis would become as rare as other vitamin deficiency diseases, such as scurvy, beriberi, pellagra and rickets."

The clinical experiments which Dr. Barton-Wright describes involved the use of other additional agents beside pantothenic acid, and the results as reported are most promising. Scientifically controlled experimental trials would be, he indicates, very expensive. Conservatively I think we would have to conclude that nobody *knows* whether or under what circumstances pantothenic acid can be used effectively against rheumatoid arthritis.[15] It needs to be tried.

A question regarding the other vitamin which is of peculiar personal interest to me is: "Are pregnant women in this country often deficient in folic acid, as has been indicated by several investigations?"[16] I doubt if we can say with certainty that we *know* the answer to this important question.

This question is important because it is well-established that when experimental animals are deficient in folic acid during various stages of pregnancy, *all sorts of malformations* occur in the offspring. Deformity of any organ or structure in the body can result, including deformities of the heart and blood vessels. If pregnant women are often even mildly deficient in folic acid knowledge of this fact can probably prevent much human suffering and save billions in hospital bills.

Questions comparable to those I have asked about pantothenic acid and folic acid can be asked by other investigators about many other nutrients with which they may be peculiarly familiar.

Interest in vitamin B_6 certainly would elicit such questions as, "What is the relationship of this vitamin to various forms of arthritis?" In spite of the extensive experience of John W. Ellis, M.D., of Mt. Pleasant, Texas, we cannot say that we *know* the answers.[17] Sufficiently controlled experiments have not been carried out. Dozens of other important questions about each of many other nutrients are still essentially unanswered, but we will not discuss these more fully here.

In some of our previous discussions, I have sought to cast doubt on the validity of the "single nutrient" approach to the treatment of disease. This approach leads to the conclusion that vitamin B_1 is for beriberi, niacinamide is for pellagra, vitamin C is for scurvy. This sounds plausible until we begin to ask what is phosphate for? What is lysine for? What is zinc for? What are the dozens of other individual nutrients for? A consideration of the futility of these questions led us to accept the teamwork principle which has been discussed earlier (p. 23).

The recognition of the teamwork principle leads us to ask a whole set of new questions, none of which has been answered because they have not been subjected to trial. Representative questions in this category are these: Can the mending of broken bones and the recovery from other injuries be hastened by the teamwork approach, giving to the individual sophisticated, well-rounded nutrition, taking into account every nutrient and the patient's individual needs? Can the development of an infant without damaging defects of any kind be *insured* by providing the prospective mother, from the start, what may be regarded, with sophistication, to be excellent nutrition? Can mental retardation be prevented by this means? Can the number of heart disease victims be decreased by furnishing excellent postnatal nutrition? Can anything be done nutritionally to prevent kidney disease and hypertension? Can the teamwork approach be used successfully to prevent and treat arthritis? Can mental disease be lessened or eliminated by providing each individual prenatally and postnatally with the best possible nutrition? Can dental disease be decreased or eliminated by the same means? How about decreasing or eliminating alcoholism by using the same strategy? Can anything be done, using the teamwork principle, to fight cancer?

It would take us too far afield if we were to enter into a discussion of the cancer problem. Cancer is one of the many diseases which has not been studied from the standpoint of sophisticated nutrition.[18] There are many hints from current investigations that there is hope in this area; not from charlatans but from serious scientific investigation.

A number of general questions related to nutrition are presently unanswered. For example, how can we find out in individual cases what the crucial nutritional needs may be? This question is a large one and would require an extensive answer. It can only come as a result of extensive experimentation and the development of automated and computerized methods.

One question of a general nature is this: Will such expedients as restriction of food intake, fasting, or avoidance of full meals, promote well-being or longevity in human beings?[19] Many studies indicate that such measures are effective with rats. Is there danger of trace element deficiencies in human nutrition? Careful experiments suggest that there is, but more detailed definitive information is needed before we can say that we *know*.[20] What relation does chelation have to this problem?

Does excellent nutrition protect against contaminants and pollutants in the air, water and food?[21] (See Ch. 10, pg. 86.) To what extent? We know in some cases that there is protection, but the answer to the general question is very incomplete.

A question not usually thought of in connection with nutrition is this: When we sleep, is there some nutrition-related building going on in our brains? Why we human beings need sleep at all is not known. There must be some very fundamental reason because we spend about a third of our life span doing it. Characteristically a human being spends many consecutive hours (it usually *seems* a short time) of "effort" before he gains his objective—a rested individual—and then after a day's activity he has it all to do over again. Whatever is accomplished during sleep is a reversible process and becomes "undone" during the period of wakefulness. There is no single sleep pattern that all do or should follow, but no one escapes a periodic *time-consuming* operation. Since so much time is involved—one, two or three hours is wholly inadequate for most of us—it seems reasonable to think that some kind of reversible biochemical construction is proceeding, and if sleep is interrupted, there is lost motion in finding the "tools" and settling down to work again. Regardless of just what is happening, the biochemical make-up of the brain of a rested person must be different from that of one who needs sleep. Otherwise sleep accomplishes nothing, and we know this cannot be true.

This speculation leads us to ask the following nutrition-related questions, the answers to which are unknown because we know so little about biochemical sleep processes: Can the effectiveness of the sleep process be impaired by deficiencies in the raw materials furnished nutritionally to the brain? Can more effective sleep be promoted by providing an excellent environment for the brain cells? Can sleep time be decreased by providing super nutrition?

We have observed in our laboratories in testing single foods as to their ability to support life, that certain foods, notably rice, do not furnish good nutrition for growth and development of young rats, yet seem to prolong life. Why? We do not know.

This leads us to ask a much broader question to which nutritional science cannot yet give adequate or definitive answers: May different diets exhibit excellence in different directions? To take an extreme case, is it possible that the best diet for promoting good body and muscle development would not be the best for promoting brain development? Could a diet be highly effective in producing *rapid* development, and yet not produce *sound* development? Can a diet be excellent for fostering reproduction but not so good for promoting longevity?

We do not even know whether these are valid or important questions. There are many reasons for entertaining, at least for the time being, the general idea that excellent prenatal and postnatal nutrition as presently conceived, foster the development of *all* faculties and pave the way for a long life. This, of course, does not preclude the desirability of modifying nutrition with advancing development and age.

According to a newspaper report appearing at the time of this writing, Dr. Ralph Nelson of the Mayo Clinic has advocated a low protein "longevity diet" for athletes.[22] Such a recommendation must be based upon opinion rather than upon knowledge because certainly no controlled experiments have ever demonstrated that such a diet (or any other diet) is optimally effective for athletes.

This leads to another question: Why do athletes, baseball pitchers, football quarterbacks, tennis players, and others have "off-days" when they can't seem to deliver? Can it be that such temporary incapacity is related to temporary failures in their nutrition, like getting too much toxicants from foods or other improprieties? The reason why this appears to be an important question is because there is hope that answers may be earnestly sought and found. Gifted professional athletes are, market-wise, highly valuable commodities, and there is an inducement to watch their nutrition as carefully as one would watch the environment of a valuable race horse like Secretariat.

Still another question which is unusual because of the restricted and underdeveloped position nutrition has maintained is as follows: Does the nutrition of test animals need to be carefully considered in connection with the testing of potential drugs? Does the nutrition of patients need to be considered in connection with the administration of drugs to them? Suppose, for example, a drug is judged to be "safe" when tested on a group of well-nourished animals. This is a prescribed routine. This drug is then administered to human beings who are, perhaps by comparison with the animals, very poorly nourished. Does this make any difference? No great difficulty arises *unless* nutrition has a substantial effect on resistance to drugs. This is probably the case. If poorly fed animals were used in testing the potential drug, the conclusion might easily have been drawn that the drug is *unsafe;* it probably would have killed too many of the animals. Drugs which are judged safe when tested on very well-nourished animals may cause death when administered to an individual in a poor nutritional state. This is not entirely speculative since we have found evidences in our laboratories recently that poorly nourished animals are distinctly less resistant to some poisons. The important point is: we do not know how important the nutritional factor may be.

A host of other "areas of ignorance" exist in the field of nutrition. In most of these areas there is no dearth of *opinion*, but a great lack of sound *knowledge*. How many patients have poor nutrition as a result of digestive or absorptive difficulties? To what extent is the intestinal flora a factor in providing needed nutrients? Can the flora be modified to make it more effective? What do we *know* about the use and abuse of "megavitamin" therapy? Can self-selection of foods under some circumstances militate *against* good health? Are the so-called "organically grown" foods appreciably superior to those grown commercially? Are the reported toxic properties of vitamin A due to contaminating impurities rather than to the vitamin itself?[23] Is coenzyme Q a nutrient involved in intercellular symbiosis?[24] Are forms of vitamin D dangerous even at lower levels of intake?[25] To what extent can nutrition be deployed to overcome or lessen stress? How is nutrition related to the broad problem of hormone production? To how great a degree is immunity or resistance to disease dependent on good nutrition? Do imbalances between nutrients (other than between amino acids or between certain common minerals) militate seriously against good nutrition? Do we place too much reliance on *rat* nutrition or should several other species be used more? Is the genetotrophic principle sound and widely applicable? Is it applicable only when certain types of heritable characteristics are involved? How is nutrition, including intercellular nutrition, related to the vast biological problem of cell differentiation? In the medical dictionary I most often use, there are over sixteen columns devoted to listing roughly 1,000 named diseases. Of these, how many are influenced or are capable of being influenced by nutritional factors?

So far in this book I have made no pleas. In conclusion, I beg your indulgence to make one urgent request. I hope those who read this book—physicians, scientists, laymen or whoever—will use their influence to help see that more serious consistent scientific attention is given to the questions that have arisen in this chapter as well as other nutrition-related problems. This implies a conservative approach which relies not on the opinions of self-styled experts but rather on the findings of investigators who seek, first-hand, to find answers to pressing problems.

REFERENCES

1. Reed, L.J., and Cox, D.J.: Macromolecular organization of enzyme systems. In *Annual Review of Biochemistry*. Palo Alto, Annual Reviews, Inc., 1966.

2. DeBusk, B.G., and Williams, R.J.: Effect of lipoic acid on the growth rate of young chicks and rats. *Arch Biochem. Biophys.*, *55*:587, 1955.

3. Mardones, R.J., et al.: Effect of synthetic thioctic acid or α lipoic acid on the voluntary alcohol intake of rats. *Science, 119*:735, 1954.

4. Schultze, M.O.: Nutrition of rats with compounds of known chemical structure. *J. Nutr., 61*:585, 1957.

5. Schneider, H.A.: Ecological ectocrines in experimental epidemiology. *Science, 158*:597, 1967.

6. Bollag, W.: Prophylaxis of chemically-inducted papillomas and carcinomas of mouse skin by vitamin A acid. *Experentia, 28*:1219, 1972.

7. Holick, M.F., et al.: 1 α hydroxy derivative of vitamin D_3: A highly potent analog. of 1 α dihydroxy vitamin D_3. *Science, 180*:190, 1973.

8. Rogers, Q.R., and Harper, A.E.: Selection of a solution containing histidine by rats fed a histidine imbalanced diet. *J. Comp. Physiol. Psychol., 72*:66, 1970.

9. Leung, P.M.B., and Rogers Q.R.: Effect of amino acid imbalance and deficiency on food intake of rats with hypothalmic lesions. *Life Sci., 8*:1, 1969.

10. Yudkin, John: *Sweet and Dangerous*. New York, Bantam, 1972.

11. Williams, R.J., Pelton, R.B., and Siegel, F.L.: Individuality as exhibited by inbred animals: Its implications for human behavior. *Proc. Natl. Acad. Sci., 48*:1461, 1962.

12. Coca, Arthur: *Pulse Test*. New York, Arc. 1968.

13. Taylor, A., Thacker, J., and Pennington, D.E.: The effect of increased pantothenic acid in the egg on the development of the embryo. *Science, 94*:542, 1941.

14. Barton-Wright, E.C.: *Arthritis: A Deficiency Disease*. London, United Trade Press, 1973.

15. Williams, R.J.: *Nutrition Against Disease*. New York, Pitman, 1971.

16. Nelson, M.M., et al.: Multiple congenital abnormalties resulting from transitory deficiency of pteroylglutamic acid during gestation in the rat. *J. Nutr., 56*:349, 1955.

17. Ellis, John, and Presley, J.: *Vitamin B_6: The Doctor's Report*. New York, Har-Row, 1973.

18. Williams, R.J.: *Nutrition Against Disease*. New York, Pitman, 1971, Ch. 12.

19. McCay, C.M.: Diet and Ageing. *Vitam. Horm.*, 7:147, 1949.

20. Schroeder, H.A.: Losses of vitamins and trace minerals resulting from processing and preservation of foods. *Am. J. Clin. Nutr., 24*:562, 1971.

21. Tappel, A.C.: Vitamin E. *Nutr. Today*, July-August, 1973.

22. Getz, George: Diet tie to life viewed. In *Los Angeles Times*, Dec. 7, 1973.

23. Vedder, E.B., and Rosenberg, C.: Concerning the toxicity of vitamin A. *J. Nutr., 16*:57, 1938.
24. Littarman, G., et al.: Evidence for a deficiency of co-enzyme Q in human heart disease. *Int. J. Vitam. Res., 40*:380, 1971.
25. Moon, J.Y.: Factors affecting steroid calcification associated with atherosclerosis. *Atherosclerosis, 16*:119, 1972.

INDEX